STEPPING STONES TO Recovery

®

ZOAR HOME
3724 Mt. Royal Boulevard
Allison Park, PA 15101
(412) 486-9400

STEPPING STONES TO Recovery

From Cocaine/Crack Addiction

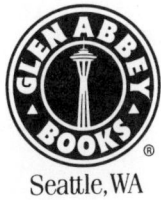

Seattle, WA

Copyright © 1990 by Anonymous

Published by Glen Abbey Books, Inc.
All rights reserved.

No part of this book may be reproduced in any form by any means without the prior written permission of the author.

Cover design by
  Graphiti Associates, Inc.
  Seattle, Washington

The 12 Steps and 12 Traditions are reprinted and adapted with permission of A.A. World Services, Inc.
  Permission to reprint and adapt the Steps and Traditions does not mean A.A. has reviewed or approved the contents of this publication nor that A.A. agrees with the views expressed herein.
  Alcoholics Anonymous is a program of recovery from alcoholism. The use of the Steps and Traditions in connection with programs and activities which are patterned after A.A. but which address other problems does not imply otherwise.

NOTE: 1. *Alcoholics Anonymous*, p. 63
       2. *Alcoholics Anonymous*, p. 76
       3. *The Connection*, Summer 1988
       4. *N.A. Way*, October 1987

First Edition
ISBN 0-934125-10-4
Printed in the United States of America

---

10 9 8 7 6 5 4 3 2 1

DEDICATED TO

The Early Members and Founders of
Cocaine Anonymous
and
Narcotics Anonymous

INTRODUCTION

When we speak of the miracle of 12 Step recovery, we are talking about people stopping their active addiction and living a better life free of addictive substances. The miracle happens when we begin our First Step and realize we are joining a group of people like ourselves, who have had similar problems but who are making it.

No matter how bad off we are when we begin 12 Step recovery—no job, no place to live, debt, legal hassles, marital or relationship problems, the list goes on—we will meet fellow members who have overcome problems like ours and are willing to help us. The miracle takes place when someone says to a newcomer, "I've been through that. Can I help you?"

Many of us needed a complete overhaul of many aspects of our lives besides stopping our cocaine, drug, and/or alcohol addiction. We found that help in our 12 Step Fellowship. The chapters in this book outline what addiction is and point the way out.

Mark R. & Mary L.

CONTENTS

INTRODUCTION

Chapter 1
COCAINE—BASIC FACTS

What Is It? 1
What It Does 1
How It Is Used 1
Why We Used It 2
Addiction 2
Am I An Addict? 3

Chapter 2
TOOLS OF RECOVERY

Abstinence 13
The 12 Steps 13
The 12 Traditions 14
Meetings 14
Reading 15
Sponsorship 16
One Day At A Time 16
Service 17
Fellow Members 17
Slogans 17
Spirituality 18
Prayer and Meditation 18

Chapter 3
WORKING THE PROGRAM

Honesty 19
Hope 21
Willingness 22
Courage 23
Truthfulness 23
Character Building 24
Humility 25
Forgiveness 25
Faith 26
Self-Examination 27
Conscious Contact 27
Service 28
Anonymity 29
Principles 29

Chapter 4
12 STEP PRAYERS AND MEDITATIONS

First Step Prayer 31
Early Recovery 31
Second Step Prayer 32
Not God 32
Third Step Prayer 33
Let Go And Let God 33
Fourth Step Prayer 33
Honesty 34
Fifth Step Prayer 34
Admitting Wrongs 35

Sixth Step Prayer 35
Defects 36
Seventh Step Prayer 36
Transformation 36
Eighth Step Prayer 37
I'm Sorry 37
Ninth Step Prayer 38
Amends 38
Tenth Step Prayer 39
Common Sense 39
Eleventh Step Prayer 40
Conscious Contact 40
Twelfth Step Prayer 41
Helping Others 41

Chapter 5
CAUTION: RELAPSE TRIGGERS

Glamorizing 43
Mistakes 44
Slippery Places and People 44
Identify, Don't Compare 45
Problems Happen 46
Stress 47
Total Abstinence 47
Dreams 48
Immaturity 48
H.A.L.T. 49
Stinking Thinking 49
Complacency 50
Boredom 50
Sex 50

Chapter 6
PERSONAL SHARING

Money	53
Accepting Myself	54
Trying To Figure It Out	54
Denial Isn't A River In Africa	55
Procrastination	56
As We Understood	58
Dating	59
The Slip	60
Gratitude	60
Willing To Change	61
Changes	64
Your Baby's A Junkie	66
Motivation	69
Letting Go	70
No More Running Away	71
Feelings	72
Never Too Young To Die	73

Chapter 7
THE PROMISES

The First Promise	78
The Second Promise	79
The Third Promise	80
The Fourth Promise	81
The Fifth Promise	82
The Sixth Promise	83
The Seventh Promise	84
The Eighth Promise	85

The Ninth Promise 86
The Tenth Promise 87
The Eleventh Promise 88
The Twelfth Promise 89

Chapter 8
SLOGANS 91

COCAINE ANONYMOUS 97

THE TWELVE STEPS
OF COCAINE ANONYMOUS 98

THE TWELVE TRADITIONS
OF COCAINE ANONYMOUS 99

THE TWELVE STEPS
OF NARCOTICS ANONYMOUS 100

THE TWELVE TRADITIONS
OF NARCOTICS ANONYMOUS 101

THE TWELVE STEPS
OF ALCOHOLICS ANONYMOUS 102

THE TWELVE TRADITIONS
OF ALCOHOLICS ANONYMOUS 103

PRAYER OF ST. FRANCIS ASSISI

*Lord, make me an instrument
of Your peace!
Where there is hatred, let me sow love.
Where there is injury, pardon.
Where there is doubt, faith.
Where there is despair, hope.
Where there is darkness, light.
Where there is sadness, joy.*

*O Divine Master,
grant that I may not so much seek
To be consoled as to console.
To be understood as to understand.
To be loved as to love.
For it is in giving
that we receive.
It is in pardoning
that we are pardoned.
It is in dying
that we are born to eternal life.*

SERENITY PRAYER

*God grant me the Serenity
To accept the things I cannot change;
Courage to change the things I can;
And Wisdom to know the difference.*

*Living one day at a time;
Enjoying one moment at a time;
Accepting hardship as the pathway to peace;*

*Taking, as He did,
this simple world as it is,
not as I would have it;
Trusting that He will
make all things right
if I surrender to His Will;*

*That I may be
reasonably happy in this life,
and supremely happy with Him
forever in the next.*

1
COCAINE—BASIC FACTS

WHAT IS IT?

We don't need to spend too much time on what cocaine is—as addicts, we know. The cocaine we have used comes to us as powder or rocks. It comes from the leaves of a plant which grows mostly in Central and South America. We didn't really care where it came from, because we knew where to get it locally. We usually didn't know how pure it was—how many times it had been stepped on. We knew it was illegal and we really didn't care.

WHAT IT DOES

Cocaine does two things: it is a local anesthetic and a central nervous system stimulant. It numbs our skin where we put it and it gives our brain a rush. It's the only drug that does both.

HOW IT IS USED

To get the effects of cocaine, one can shoot it, snort it, or smoke it.

WHY WE USED IT

The reasons we used, as well as the way we were introduced to cocaine, are different for everyone. As recovering addicts, we won't tell you we never thought using cocaine was wonderful. At first we liked it, then we fell in love with it, then it tried to kill us. How did we go from the pleasure to the pain?

ADDICTION

We didn't start out to become addicts. During our early use, we thought the warnings, "the big lie," etc., were funny. We didn't buy any of that. How could something be illegal and bad for you when it felt so good?

This was because nothing bad had happened to us "yet." As cocaine began to take control of our bodies, minds, and behavior, we denied more and more that it was harmful.

We really don't understand what it's like to be an occasional user of cocaine—someone who can take it and leave it alone. It was difficult for us to admit, finally, that we had a disease, that we were out of control. For those of us now in 12 Step recovery, we each have a different but similar story on how we became willing to live without mood-altering chemicals. We each have a different story about what got us the help we need.

We were not very happy when we looked at our addiction and thought of stopping. We were angry with the police, the courts, friends, family, doctors, or employers who made us face our addiction. We were the last ones to find out we were addicts. We were like the operator of a huge searchlight. We shone the spotlight on everything and everybody else before we put the beam on ourselves and took responsibility for finding a way out.

How did we finally discover we were addicts? That we had a disease which was doing everything to tell us we didn't have it? Many of us got the help and information at an in-patient or out-patient treatment facility, through 12 Step members, counselors, or therapists.

Many times, the information about addiction, chemical dependency, alcoholism, or whatever name fits, came in the following ways.

Many of us took this "yes or no" test. The word "cocaine" can be replaced with "drug" or "alcohol" or what fits for you.

AM I AN ADDICT?

	Yes	No
1. Do you lose time from work or school due to your cocaine use?	❑	❑
2. Do you use cocaine alone?	❑	❑
3. Is your cocaine use making your home life unhappy?	❑	❑
4. Have you ever switched from one drug to another, thinking if you stop the drug that's giving you problems, you'll be O.K.?	❑	❑
5. Do you use cocaine because you're shy with other people?	❑	❑
6. Is your drug use affecting your reputation (have others lost respect for you)?	❑	❑

	Yes	No
7. Have you ever lied, conned, or manipulated a doctor to give you a prescription?	☐	☐
8. Have you stolen drugs?	☐	☐
9. Have you done anything illegal to get money for drugs?	☐	☐
10. Have you felt guilty or ashamed after drug use?	☐	☐
11. Has drug use caused financial difficulties?	☐	☐
12. Have you mixed other drugs or alcohol with cocaine to get a better buzz?	☐	☐
13. Have you used other drugs or alcohol to get over cocaine hangovers?	☐	☐
14. Do you use cocaine to get you going in the morning?	☐	☐
15. Do you hang out with people or go to places that could be dangerous?	☐	☐
16. Do you sometimes think you're crazy?	☐	☐
17. Has cocaine put you, your friends, or your loved ones in unhealthy situations?	☐	☐
18. Do you crave cocaine at a certain time of the day?	☐	☐
19. Has cocaine gotten you in trouble with the law?	☐	☐
20. Has your ambition or efficiency decreased because of your cocaine use?	☐	☐
21. Do you see or hear things that aren't real?	☐	☐

FROM COCAINE/CRACK

	Yes	No
22. Has cocaine affected your relationships or marriage?	❏	❏
23. Have you ever minimized or denied your drug use when asked?	❏	❏
24. Does cocaine interfere with eating or sleeping?	❏	❏
25. Have you experienced blackouts or loss of memory?	❏	❏
26. Has cocaine affected your sex life negatively?	❏	❏
27. Have you seen a doctor or been in a hospital or treatment center because of cocaine use?	❏	❏
28. Do you keep using cocaine even though your life is going in the toilet?	❏	❏
29. Do you use cocaine to escape from stress, worry, troubles, or responsibility?	❏	❏
30. Have you ever tried to quit using cocaine and couldn't stop?	❏	❏
31. Have you overdosed or gotten sick from using cocaine?	❏	❏
32. Do you always think about getting and using cocaine?	❏	❏
33. Does cocaine make you paranoid?	❏	❏
34. Do you stay away from people and places that don't approve of your cocaine use?	❏	❏
35. Do you believe you are a cocaine addict?	❏	❏

We were told if we answered "yes" to too many of these questions, we were addicts. But we were the only ones who could make the choice of whether or not we believed it. These questions showed us we had a problem and our lives were out of control.

The *Diagnostic and Statistical Manual* (DSM-111-R) of the American Psychiatric Association lists specific behaviors and signs of cocaine addiction. If a person shows three or more of the following, they have a problem:

1. Cocaine is often taken in large amounts or over a longer period of time than the user intended.
2. The user has a persistent desire, or has made one or more unsuccessful attempts to cut down or control his/her cocaine use.
3. The user spends a great deal of time in activities necessary to obtain cocaine, use cocaine, or recover from its effects.
4. The user is frequently intoxicated or experiencing post-drug reactions when expected to fulfill major role obligations at work, school, or home, or when cocaine use is physically hazardous (e.g., driving a car while high on cocaine).
5. The user foregoes important social, occupational, or recreational activities because of cocaine use.
6. The user continues to take cocaine despite the knowledge that persistent or recurrent social, psychological, or physical problems are being caused or exacerbated by the continued use.
7. The user shows marked tolerance to cocaine evidenced by the need for substantially increased amounts of the drug in order to achieve intoxication or other desired effects, or shows a markedly diminished effect from continued use of the same amount.

We also learn about cocaine addiction by reviewing the definition of alcoholism from the American Society of Addiction Medicine, and the National Council on Alcoholism and Drug Dependence:

Definition of Alcoholism

Alcoholism is a **primary**, chronic **disease** with genetic, psychosocial, and environmental factors influencing its development and manifestations. The disease is **often progressive and fatal.** It is characterized by continuous or periodic **impaired control** over drinking, **preoccupation** with the drug alcohol, use of alcohol despite **adverse consequences**, and distortions in thinking, most notably **denial.**

- **primary** refers to the nature of alcoholism as a disease entity in addition to and separate from other pathophysiologic states which may be associated with it. **Primary** suggests that alcoholism, as an addiction, is not a symptom of an underlying disease state.

- **disease** means an involuntary disability. It represents the sum of the abnormal phenomena displayed by a group of individuals. These phenomena are associated with a specified common set of characteristics by which these individuals differ from the norm, and which places them at a disadvantage.

- **often progressive and fatal** means that the disease persists over time and that physical, emotional, and social changes are often cumulative and may progress as drinking continues. Alcoholism causes premature death through overdose, organic complications involving the brain, liver, heart and many other organs, and by contributing to suicide, homicide, motor vehicle crashes, and other traumatic events.

- **impaired control** means the inability to limit alcohol use or to consistently limit on any drinking occasion the duration of the episode, the quantity consumed, and/or the behavioral consequences of drinking.

- **preoccupation** in association with alcohol use indicates excessive, focused attention given to the drug alcohol, its effects, and/or its use. The relative value thus assigned to alcohol by the individual often leads to a diversion of energies away from important life concerns.

- **adverse consequences** are alcohol-related problems or impairments in such areas as: physical health (e.g., alcohol withdrawal syndromes, liver disease, gastritis, anemia, neurological disorders); psychological functioning (e.g., impairments in cognition, changes in mood and behavior); interpersonal functioning (e.g., marital problems and child abuse, impaired social relationships); occupational functioning (e.g., scholastic or job problems); and legal, financial, or spiritual problems.

- **denial** is used here not only in the psychoanalytic sense of a single psychological defense mechanism disavowing the significance of events, but more broadly to include a range of psychological maneuvers designed to reduce awareness of the fact that alcohol use is the cause of an individual's problems rather than a solution to those problems. **Denial** becomes an integral part of the disease and a major obstacle to recovery.

(*This definition was prepared by the Joint Committee to Study the Definition and Criteria for the Diagnosis of Alcoholism of the National Council on Alcoholism and Drug Dependence and the American Society of Addiction Medicine. It was approved by the Board of Directors of NCADD on 3 February, 1990 and the Board of Directors of ASAM on 25 February, 1990.* **Prevention Pipeline 3(3), May/June 1990.**)

Another way to understand what cocaine addiction **is**, is to list what it **is not**.

1. Cocaine addiction is a disease like diabetes, cancer, or AIDS. It is not an illness like a toothache, headache, or upset stomach.
2. Cocaine addiction creates problems; it is not caused by them. It is not caused by a job, financial difficulties, or family problems.
3. Cocaine addiction is not freedom; it controls those addicted to it.
4. Cocaine addiction is chronic and progressive (it keeps getting worse). It is not just about getting into fights, getting arrested, or the bad things it does to our minds and bodies.
5. Cocaine addiction is characterized by "loss of control" over how much and when we use it. It doesn't necessarily mean we use all the time. Even when we stay away from cocaine for a while, when we start again we "lose control."
6. Cocaine addiction can be treated at any point. One does not have to lose everything to begin recovery.
7. Cocaine addiction is a disease. Why we have it is not as important as knowing it can be stopped and treated.

8. Cocaine addiction means not only staying abstinence from cocaine, but staying abstinent from all mood-altering drugs, including alcohol.

It is important to get the facts about addiction and admit that we are addicts. This is the starting point. Most of us knew we were addicts and in trouble with our drug use before the significant event which brought us to seek help. The help that we outline in this book is the 12 Step recovery program found in A.A. (Alcoholics Anonymous), N.A. (Narcotics Anonymous), D.A. (Drugs Anonymous), or C.A. (Cocaine Anonymous).

We, the authors, each came at our recovery from a different direction:

My name is Mark, and I'm an alcoholic. My recovery program is A.A. because alcohol was my drug of choice. All the other drugs I used were in addition to my alcohol use. I think of it as alcohol being the sun and the other drugs I used as the planets revolving around the sun. It wasn't until I got into cocaine that I really hit bottom. So my recovery has been in A.A. I don't talk about cocaine at meetings because I have put all other drugs into one—alcohol. I'm comfortable doing it this way, and I don't step on anyone's toes in A.A. talking about cocaine.

My name is Mary and I am an addict. I have found recovery in C.A. from my cocaine addiction. Cocaine was my drug of choice and C.A. meetings and friends have helped me the most. Both Mark and myself have found the 12 Step program that fits for us. Some go to N.A. or go to meetings of different fellowships, but remember to respect the boundaries of each fellowship.

The next chapters will outline the basic parts of 12 Step recovery that are common to all anonymous organizations.

2
TOOLS OF RECOVERY

All anonymous fellowships are based on the ideas of Alcoholics Anonymous, which was founded in 1935. Narcotics Anonymous was founded in 1953, and Cocaine Anonymous was founded in 1982.

N.A. and C.A. received permission from A.A. to adapt the Preamble, 12 Steps, and 12 Traditions to their specific program. We have reprinted these at the end of this book. There are parts of each organization that are basic. These are often referred to as the Tools of Recovery, as follows:

ABSTINENCE

Total abstinence from all mood-altering addictive substances. If we want to stay off cocaine, we stop all other drugs as well. We can't switch from cocaine to pot, for instance.

THE 12 STEPS

The first three Steps show us how to **give up**. Steps 4, 5, and 6 teach us how to **own up**. Steps 7, 8, and 9 teach us how to **make up**. Steps 10, 11, and 12 teach us how to **grow up**. Each Step must be worked if the program is to be effective. We are encouraged to do them in order. A two-Stepper is someone who just practices the First and Twelfth Steps and misses all the others. We hear from members that there are "12 Steps in the ladder" to continued recovery.

Can a person work just a few Steps and leave the rest? Can we just "sort of" do a Fourth Step, like in our minds? Do we really have to write it down as we're instructed? Can we do our Fifth Step with our dog or cat or a favorite tree? Can we make amends in our minds? Can we have someone else make amends for us? Do we have to do all these Steps? We feel much better about our lives now that we are in recovery, but we really can't do some of these Steps because they're too hard.

Our common experience has shown us that those who don't work all the Steps don't make it. Those that do work all the Steps do make it. We need to work the Steps in order and to the best of our ability based on our willingness and open-mindedness.

THE 12 TRADITIONS

The 12 Steps tell us **how** the program works. The Traditions tell us **why** it works. A.A. was in operation for over 10 years before the Traditions were written in the late 1940s. The success of 12 Step fellowships is based on the wisdom in the Traditions.

MEETINGS

We are told at first that we **have to** go to meetings. We find out after awhile that we **want to** go. At first we're asked to go to meetings whether we find them good or bad. We just go. We find meetings we enjoy and then select a home group.

We hear from those who have been in recovery for awhile that there really are no bad meetings. All meetings are good; some are just better than others. We are reminded to "bring the body and the mind will follow," and "take what you need and leave the rest."

Even when we think we didn't get much out of a meeting, we will find that many others who were there benefited a great deal. We may remember something we heard at a "bad" meeting more often than what we heard at a "good" meeting. The old-timers tell us, "The most important part of any meeting, for you, is the moment you walk through the door into it. It's not so much what you do there; it's the fact that you are there."

Meetings are not the means to an end. Meetings are an end in themselves, a way of life. Each meeting is it's own reward. We hear people talk of a meeting being one stone in the foundation of recovery. If we have accumulated many of these stones, when temptation comes our way we will have built a good foundation to say no. Since we are never cured, we remember that "When we want to go to a meeting, we can walk. When we don't, we should run."

READING

We all benefit from reading. There are many good books and pamphlets available for us to read. The knowledge we gain from reading helps us understand ourselves and our world better. The fogginess and lack of concentration we have when we first begin recovery fades away. Reading and the wisdom of books helps us on our journey of recovery.

SPONSORSHIP

Before we are in the program very long it is suggested we find a sponsor. We find a person who has the kind of recovery we want. The reason for finding a sponsor is to have someone who can guide us through the 12 Steps and help us apply them to problems we encounter.

Sponsorship is one of the important ways of carrying the message. Sponsors freely share their experience of working the program. They don't nag or manage our lives. At times, sponsors may appear strict, but they're only passing on their knowledge. They have a deep concern about us and our recovery.

Sponsors listen to us and give us suggestions. They tell us what has worked for them, point out possible trouble spots, and help us decide what to do about them. Sponsors help us understand the program, and guide us along the path of recovery.

We find a sponsor by asking the group secretary if there is a temporary sponsor sign-up sheet, or by raising our hand at a meeting and asking for a temporary sponsor. After a time in recovery we too become sponsors and help those who are newcomers.

No matter how long we have been clean and sober, we still need a sponsor. It is a vital part of the program.

ONE DAY AT A TIME

Twelve Step recovery is a "one-day-at-a-time" way of living. Life is easier to handle broken up into manageable pieces. We deal with our addiction for 24-hour periods. When we're new, we may be hanging in there an hour, or even a minute, at a time. We do our work one task at a time. We solve our problems one at a time.

When we live in the now, for this day only, one day at a time, we assure ourselves a comfortable reality.

SERVICE

We become less concerned about ourselves in recovery. We learn to be of service to others. Service can take the form of setting up chairs for meetings, making coffee, or taking someone to a meeting. One of the paradoxes of the program is that in order to grow and keep our recovery, we need to be of service to others and pass on what we've been given. When we give away what we've learned, we are keeping it.

Many of us become involved in the service structure of our individual group or fellowship. Some become active in the organizational aspects of the fellowship.

FELLOW MEMBERS

We find friends in recovery. We realize we are no longer alone. We discover we are people who need people. We unlearn our addictive ways of using people. Our program suggests we work for recovery for ourselves, but we can't do it alone. None of us need to ever be alone again. We are bound together by a common problem and work together for solutions.

SLOGANS

Live and Let Live, Easy Does It, But For The Grace Of God, Think, Think, Think, and First Things First—these are the slogans we most often hear and see on the walls of our meeting rooms. There is another popular slogan which is an acronym of the first words of these five slogans: "Live Easy But Think First."

Many newcomers hear that we begin recovery on the slogans and stay in recovery on the 12 Steps. The slogans were developed for use in recovery from the experience of many others. At first, they may appear too simple (and sometimes too corny) for us to use. The slogans are anything but corny. We need to check if we are using them in our daily lives.

SPIRITUALITY

Twelve Step recovery has to do with spirituality, not religion. We come to the spiritual through our discovery of a power **other** than ourselves. We learn to give up playing God and trying to control everything and everyone around us. This Power is not something over which we have any control. We can only identify it as greater than we are. As we work the Steps, our experience with our own Higher Power grows. We start to trust the influence this Power has over our lives. Many of us feel comfortable calling this Power God. Some even continue their journey back into a particular religion. Each person in recovery comes to terms with their own spirit life in their own way.

PRAYER AND MEDITATION

These are two very valuable tools in recovery. Prayer and meditation help us stay connected to our Higher Power. In prayer, we seek answers and direction in life. In meditation, we listen for answers. Step prayers and meditations are reprinted in Chapter 4.

3
WORKING THE PROGRAM

Our success in the Program, our level of happiness in recovery, our overall attitude about living without drugs is decided by how hard we work for it. We will get from the Steps only as much as we give. The rewards we receive from the program are equal to the effort we put into our recovery. The following are the different parts of the program and "why it works."

HONESTY

The First Step asks us to be honest with ourselves. Are we powerless over cocaine? Has it made our life unmanageable? Honesty is vital to our recovery. It has to begin within us and must flow outward from us. To be true to ourselves, we can't think one thing and do another. When we were using, our denial spelled dishonesty. So did the false fronts we put up to impress others.

Dishonesty was motivated by fear and our low self-esteem. We hated ourselves, and we were afraid others would hate us too, if we showed them honestly who we were. So we lied to them and to ourselves, trying to be the person we thought other people wanted us to be.

We felt we were living behind hundreds of masks. We tried to put the world together through our own manipulations. In recovery, we learn to like the person we are. We have no more reason to lie or put up false fronts.

We were always whole and complete. It was our dishonesty and rationalizations that made us feel small as we lived our lives in a drug-induced haze. When we honestly look at our life now and stay accountable for our actions, we put our identity back together. Honesty keeps us in the present reality and opens the door to a new future. We never have to hide again.

After we're in recovery for a time, we see that there is victory in our surrender to powerlessness. When we were using, did we ever admit anything without leaving ourselves a way out? Did we once unconditionally surrender and admit we were absolutely licked? How many times did we reach the end of the road and pretend it really wasn't? Why did it seem that enough was never enough for us? If there was any more pain or misery to be squeezed out of our lives, we seemed compelled to do so. What was it that held us back from a firm and final admission of our powerlessness over our addiction?

Finally, when we were flat on our backs, we heard ourselves say, "This is, indeed, the bottom." It was then and only then that we made our First Step admission, a surrender that the time had finally come to give it all up. At first, this admission seemed like the worst possible defeat. We have come to realize it was the beginning of the greatest victory.

HOPE

There are many gifts for us in recovery, but no gift is as wonderful as hope. Before we took our First and Second Steps, hope was nothing more than a dream. We hoped for things we didn't need. All our hoping did while we were using was drive a wedge between ourselves and reality. The program teaches us that when we stray from reality, we stray from the very things that will help us.

Each Step draws us closer to claiming the full benefits available to everyone in recovery. When we hope for a life where we know what is good and bad for us, it happens. When we hope for a new life in recovery, our hope becomes connected to our Higher Power's will for us. The hope we have is knowing that our Higher Power, fellow members, and the program are doing for us what we couldn't do for ourselves.

Many of us used to scream, "I wish I were dead!" Our addictions and crazy behavior made us hate ourselves. We didn't care if we lived or died. We hoped that life after death would give us rest from our constant battle with compulsions. Today we have found a better answer.

There is life **before** death. Those of us who once said, "Nobody cares," have found loving, caring friends who share our problems and help us find the answers. They guide us daily through wonderful adventures of growth. We all receive great truths in recovery. We have been given the chance to live two lives. The cruel one has gone. The second one is rich with blessings.

Our old world of an out-of-control self-will was bizarre and irrational. Everything was turned around: right was left, up was down, good was bad, white was black, night was day. We could trust in nothing, because nothing trusted us. We believed in no one because no one believed in us. We loved nothing because we thought nothing loved us. We became cruel and mean-spirited. We lived life always on the defensive.

The more we acted on the strength of our own ego, the smaller our world became. Finally, in desperation, we shut everyone and everything out. Then we were truly isolated, living in a make-believe world filled with dragons, monsters, and ghosts. Our craziness had painted us into a corner and our lives were in the toilet.

We learn in recovery that the way to stop our craziness is our Second Step. Our sanity has been restored. We no longer keep repeating the same crazy mistakes, expecting different results.

WILLINGNESS

In the program we use the simple slogan H.O.W. = **H**onesty, **O**pen-mindedness, **W**illingness. This is the key we need to open up the door and begin the Third Step. We approach all challenges with honest intentions and open-minded tolerance, but only willingness will start us toward goals. Our Third Step decision is based on our willingness to live a different and happier life.

When the willingness is great, the difficulties cannot be great. If we are willing to accept and to act with dedication, nothing can stop us as long as our goals are realistic. Willingness may simply mean we are ready and well-prepared to face challenges. However, we must be cautious not to mistake **willful** for **willing**. The first insists that things happen our way and on our time schedule. The second rids us of fears and prepares us to choose wisely. We are told one of the essentials of recovery is the belief that "willingness without action is fantasy."

COURAGE

One word often heard around the program is "will." Yet, the will to do something cannot exist without the action required to do it, and that takes courage. Our Fourth Step asks us to have courage as we do our written inventory. It is courage that turns possibilities into realities. Experience teaches us that courage keeps our active emotions under control.

When courage guides our honest efforts, we can be sure that we will not only be capable of succeeding, but we will be worthy of it. We learn that courage is not recklessness; it is common sense, the kind the Serenity Prayer teaches us. When we know that a goal is worth going for, courage has judgment and carefulness as allies, even though we may be moving against the tide of popular opinion or belief. We overcome our fears about setting and working toward goals. It helps us to remember, "courage is fear that has said its prayers."

TRUTHFULNESS

The Fifth Step asks us to speak truth to ourselves, others, and our Higher Power. Truth is the foundation of all knowledge and honest progress. It is the standard by which all our actions are judged. Truth can never be bought. There is no middle ground in truth. All things are either true or false.

We learn that accepting and admitting the truth helps us. It is more painful to live a lie than go through the act of telling the truth. Unless an activity begins with truth, it will be impossible to progress successfully. The advice "truth or silence" warns us of possible harm caused by hurriedly made statements.

Love and kindness must accompany truth even if we, as the giver or receiver, are pained by the truth. Our program teaches us that truth can do no more than present things as they really exist. To work our program successfully, we must always work from a foundation of truth. The Fourth and Fifth Steps educate us in applying that truth to our lives.

CHARACTER REBUILDING

We're not born with character. We have to build it through patience, self-esteem, and humility. Character is never revealed by what we think or say, no matter how wise our thoughts or words may be sometimes. Character is what we are underneath all the defensive layers we show the world.

We come into the fellowship with defective characters. Some believe our character development stopped when we started using addictive substances. Our defects of character need to be worked on. We begin with our Sixth Step. We work hardest on the defects we once thought were good, such as our rebelliousness.

Character is an outer show of an inner glow that reaches others or pleases ourselves. It is a reserve force for all of us. Its usefulness goes beyond talent. Its greatest energy comes from personal relationships with others. Character permits us to welcome healthy criticism. It is a force that respects truth and develops willingness and spirit. It is positive. It stresses action and makes all of these clear to others.

In recovery, we examine our character and learn to develop it with patience, self-esteem, and humility.

HUMILITY

The Seventh Step asks us to be humble. We have all had our own idea of what humility is. In recovery we learn a new definition: humility is not thinking less of yourself, but thinking of yourself less. Our first ideas of humility were based on the notion we were supposed to accept anything that came our way, however humiliating. True humility doesn't mean a meek surrender to an ugly, destructive way of life. It means surrender to the realities of life and the will of our Higher Power. Humility and humiliation are two entirely different things.

Being humble is being teachable. It means staying **right size**. Humility opens us to growth in ways of living a healthy and productive life. Through humility, we gain more faith, trust, hope, helpfulness, forgiveness, charity, and the ability to freely care and share.

The simple acts of gratitude, listening, and sharing help us to cut through grandiosity and lead us toward growth in humility. When we practice humility, we are growing in strength, working on our character defects, and making spiritual progress.

FORGIVENESS

Forgiveness is an important part of our fellowship. The Eighth Step starts us on the process of forgiving others and (as importantly) ourselves. However, we are cautioned that if we forgive but don't forget we are not really practicing forgiveness.

The act of forgiveness is to bring relationships whole again wherever possible. Forgiveness is not a state of mind. It is a state of being. If we do not forgive within our hearts, we have not really forgiven. Forgiveness which stays in the head is only the intention to forgive.

We know we haven't truly forgiven when we can't forget what caused our resentments. If the wound is still open and sore, we did not forgive from the heart. We remember to give ourselves time, talk to our sponsor and fellow members, and pray for help. Finally, we have the willingness to wait. Our Higher Power will heal the wound in time. If we are willing to let go, we will be given the power to truly forgive.

FAITH

We express our faith in our program and our Higher Power during our Ninth Step amends. The Ninth Step allows us to close circles which have been open too long. Finally, we can take the "if onlies" of our lives and make the necessary amends, including those to ourselves. Those amends we cannot make directly, we ask our Higher Power to make for us.

The faith we find in our program allows us to see that we're not perfect people. We have faults. The reality we lived under the influence of cocaine told us we were more than we were. In the middle of our imperfection, our faith in the program allows us to see we are forgiven, loved, and filled with hope.

SELF-EXAMINATION

The Tenth Step reminds us to continue our inventory-taking even after our Fourth and Fifth Step housecleaning. Our world is not changing, but we know we are. When we take our daily inventory, we don't count the things we've accumulated or will accumulate; we count the times we have been on the beam or off the beam. Is our behavior more mature? Are we growing in the program?

Our daily self-examination allows us to keep our minds open and not let the garbage of procrastination and resentment build up. We end our daily inventory with gratitude to our Higher Power and the program for one more day of freedom from our disease.

CONSCIOUS CONTACT

We practice the Eleventh Step with prayer and meditation. Before we entered the program, we were always bargaining with God. "Oh God, help me! If you get me out of this mess, I'll never screw up again!" was our favorite prayer.

We have learned new prayers and a new way to talk with and listen to our Higher Power. We are seeking God's will for us. Many of us had to learn how to pray. We began very simply: "God, help me know Your will for me today." "Thank you, God, for helping me today."

We find prayer helps us with our faulty dependence on people, places, and things by giving us the insight and strength to rearrange our priorities. Trying to pray **is** praying. Prayer doesn't change God, but it changes those who pray.

We also improve our conscious contact with our Higher Power when we meditate. During meditation, we are giving ourselves time to digest the rich rewards we're finding in the program. We begin our day with a quiet time of prayer, meditation, and reflection. We take the time at night to review our day, to see the things we might improve, to remember the things we did well and enjoy them.

Meditation is a quiet time in a noisy world. It is a chance to talk with our Higher Power and to listen for answers to our questions. It's an opportunity in the evening to let stress and tension flow away, and to regain serenity. Meditation is a time of healing.

SERVICE

Our Twelfth Step encourages us to be of service to those in and out of our fellowship. Any act of "carrying the message" can serve a useful purpose, whether or not we see the results. Our home group carries the message and gives us opportunities for service.

If we maintain an attitude of being of service with love, we can work wonders at any time and every moment of the day. Through our 12 Step program, we become aware that we have the opportunity of being an example of happy, joyous, and free living without the crutch of our addiction. This "face" we present can be a positive model for anyone who comes in contact with us.

No effort must ever seem so great that it stops us from helping someone else find the kind of life we were helped to find. It is the responsibility of each member to go to any lengths in giving service. Whatever sacrifice may be required of us will bring great rewards. We learn, in the act of one person helping another, that no person can give without receiving, or get without giving. We learn from our sponsor and fellow members that when they help us, they are also helping themselves.

ANONYMITY

When we keep the principle of anonymity always in our minds, we are observing one of the most basic principles of our program. We are cautioned never to place personalities before principles. No head is higher or lower at our meetings than any other. We share the common bond of staying away from our addiction.

PRINCIPLES

The longer we are on the program, the more we enrich all parts of our lives. There is hardly a topic mentioned that does not allow us to learn. It is not that we become progressively dumber in recovery; it is just that we become progressively more open-minded. We seem to be hungry for growth opportunities.

We're not timid about meeting new people and taking part in new recovery experiences. When we have an opportunity to share our experience, strength, and hope, we do so with gratitude and humility. We can't be arrogant about our progress. We know that false pride is dangerous for us. Others have taken too much credit for their recovery and lost it.

When we practice these principles, we acknowledge our powerlessness, and our belief and trust in our

Higher Power. We keep a clear, clean conscience. We talk with our sponsors, maintain a willingness to change, and have a humble attitude. We maintain a daily inventory, pray and meditate, attend meetings, and pass it on.

4
12 STEP PRAYERS AND MEDITATIONS

FIRST STEP PRAYER

Today, I ask for help with my addiction. Denial has kept me from seeing how powerless I am and how my life is unmanageable. I need to learn and remember that I have an incurable illness and that abstinence is the only way to deal with it.

EARLY RECOVERY

Spirituality is the ability to get our minds off ourselves.
—Anonymous

The early days of recovery were a strange time for us. We were used to a very different lifestyle. There were so many new things coming into our lives all at once. Everything was whirling. We stuck close to our sponsor and home group. We needed a touchstone to make sense out of what was happening.

The early days of recovery were times of physical healing. We knew we are sick. Some of us didn't realize how sick we were. We went slow and kept our eyes, our minds, and our hearts focused on our First Step.

We didn't find instant spirituality in those days. That was O.K. There would be time enough for that;

first, we had to get started. After time on the Program, after we had worked some Steps, we were asked to get our minds off ourselves. This was the time when we started making progress with our spiritual lives.

I have learned that spirituality is the ability to get my mind off myself.

SECOND STEP PRAYER

I pray for an open mind so I may come to believe in a Power greater than myself. I pray for humility and the continued opportunity to increase my faith. I don't want to be crazy any more.

NOT GOD

First of all, we had to quit playing God. It didn't work.
—Big Book

The game we always lose is the game of playing God. When we attempt to take absolute control over either our own lives or the life of another, we only harm ourselves or them. When we inflict our own will on a situation, all we reveal is our own fear and insecurity.

Our Second Step reminds us that most of our problems have been of our own making. Until we quit trying to control everyone and everything, we could find no peace. As we work the Program with the belief that we're not God, today and tomorrow are far less frightening.

Many of us have been helped with the problem of grandiose thinking by the familiar slogan, "I can't, God can, I think I'll let Him."

Today I'll remember that if I try to play God, I'm crazy.

THIRD STEP PRAYER

God, I offer myself to Thee, to build with me and to do with me as Thou wilt. Relieve me of the bondage of self, that I may better do Thy will. Take away my difficulties, that victory over them may bear witness to those I would help of Thy Power, Thy Love, and Thy Way of life. May I do Thy will always![1]

LET GO AND LET GOD

WILL POWER = Our WILL-ingness to use a HIGHER POWER. —Anonymous

One of the greatest decisions any of us ever made concerned our Third Step. This decision seemed to go against everything we wanted to do. We all know so well that every time we tried to manage our own lives, we produced misery and heartache. Human beings seem created to fight the decision to give up control. Yet this decision in Step Three, very hard for us to make, was one of the greatest decisions we ever made.

When we did our Third Step, we merely embraced the truth. When we decided to let God be God, we were able to participate in the plan. Whenever we let go and let God, we become a player on a team that will always win.

When what I knew in the past was mostly failure, the decision to let God's will become mine continues to make sense.

FOURTH STEP PRAYER

Dear God,
It is I who have made my life a mess. I have done it, but I cannot undo it. My mistakes are mine, and I

will begin a searching and fearless moral inventory. I will write down my wrongs, but I will also include that which is good. I pray for the strength to complete the task.

HONESTY

The 12 Step way of life is honest, not necessarily self-righteous. —Anonymous

When we allowed ourselves to drift from the real world, it was often a difficult experience to find a way back. It caused deep pain and guilt. When we confronted our life history in our Fourth Step, we found that we had to go back to the very beginning to find our way home. The trip wasn't easy, but it had to be made if we were to get on with our lives.

After we began cleaning up the wreckage of our past, we made every effort to be honest daily. Now, inventory taking is gentle, with soft edges. We remember how hard it was for us to come clean and we have sympathy for those who still face this test. We guard against being righteous in our dealings with others. We do not want to wear our honesty on our sleeves. We should not be proud that we have become honest. Honesty should be as natural for us as breathing.

When I am self-righteous in my approach to others, I am not being honest; I am just being mean.

FIFTH STEP PRAYER

Higher Power, my inventory has shown me who I am, yet I ask for Your help in admitting my wrongs to another person and to You. Assure me, and be with me, in this Step, for without this Step I cannot progress in my recovery. With Your help, I can do this, and I will do it.

ADMITTING WRONGS

A man should never be ashamed to own he has been in the wrong, which is but saying, in other words, that he is wiser today than he was yesterday. —Alexander Pope

No one can grow spiritually until they have cleared their conscience and gained the respect and forgiveness of others by admitting their wrongs. Only by wiping the slate clean can we free ourselves of the constant painful reminders of acts and words which have left us with regrets, guilt, and shame. Of course, we can't be free of thoughts about the past until we have learned, through thorough inventories, the nature of our mistakes.

Our admission of wrongdoing may help others understand us better, but the person most benefited from the admission is us. The process of admitting wrongs assures us that we have accepted honesty as an asset we need in our new way of life.

The sooner I admit my mistakes, the easier they are to correct. Let me promptly admit it when I am wrong.

SIXTH STEP PRAYER

Dear God,
I am ready for Your help in removing from me the defects of character which I now realize are an obstacle to my recovery. Help me to continue being honest with myself and guide me toward spiritual and mental health.

DEFECTS

The greatest of all faults, I should say, is to be conscious of none. —Pliny

One of the first things we heard in our Program was that we probably had defects of character. We first admitted we were powerless over a substance or behavior. Then we learned that those who believed they had no faults of character were mistaken. Little progress could be made without looking at our defects of character.

Such a self-analysis, in order to be thorough, must include assets. But the big challenge is to understand our faults and to use the other Steps of the Program to get rid of them. We are not, never were, and never will be candidates for sainthood. We never try to be perfect, but give continual attention to character growth.

By doing my inventory on a daily basis, I make myself aware of my character defects and what I need to do to grow out of them.

SEVENTH STEP PRAYER

My Creator, I am willing that You should have all of me, good and bad. I pray that You now remove from me every single defect of character which stands in the way of my usefulness to You and my fellows. Grant me strength, as I go out from here to do Your bidding.[2]

TRANSFORMATION

Progress is a nice word. But change is its motivator. — Robert F. Kennedy

We humbly ask God in our Seventh Step to remove

our shortcomings. We are asking God to do in other parts of our lives what he has done to our addiction. We are a daily witness to this Power. Each moment we experience freedom from our disease, we acknowledge God's Power. Many of us lost our desire for our addiction quickly. Others waged a long and painful battle to reach a point of surrender. How will God work on our shortcomings? Will it be immediate or will it be over time?

Our Fellowship suggests that we live our lives one day at a time. Personal change occurs but one day at a time. We must resist the temptation to set God's clock to fast forward. The long-sought-after changes will occur in ways we cannot predict and should not expect.

I have not been the best judge as to what is good for me. I must trust God in all things, even those that are most personal to me.

EIGHTH STEP PRAYER

Higher Power, I ask Your help in making my list of all those I have harmed. I will take responsibility for my mistakes, and be forgiving to others as You are forgiving to me. Grant me the willingness to begin my restitution. This I pray.

I'M SORRY

The prayer of amends must be a way of life, not just a sad cry at the end of failure. —Anonymous

Most of us are truly sorry for the wreckage we caused by our behavior. Our disease has touched many people and the scars sometimes run deep. It would be great if everyone we harmed would accept our apology, but this probably won't happen. It doesn't matter. We still need to tell them we feel bad about their pain.

It's true that we offer amends in the hope of healing relationships. But it is even truer that our recovery depends on our *willingness* to offer amends. Some things can't be set right with an "I'm sorry." We have to show by *actions* as well as *words* that we honestly want to make amends where possible.

As long as I pursue my recovery one day at a time, I will have time enough to demonstrate in action that I am sorry for the pain I caused.

NINTH STEP PRAYER

Higher Power, I pray for the right attitude to make my amends, being ever mindful not to harm others in the process. I ask for Your guidance in making indirect amends. Most important, I will continue to make amends by staying abstinent, helping others, and growing in spiritual progress.

AMENDS

The first step in overcoming mistakes is to admit them.
—*Anonymous*

Amends for us are basically honest apologies of the deepest and most sincere kind. We ask not only for forgiveness from others but from ourselves as well. As we forgive, we grow spiritually. We are aware of the unkindnesses we performed and the unhappiness we heaped not only on those we thought we disliked but many whom we loved. We realize the potential for hurting others contained in our acts and words.

Sending a note or making a phone call may not be

enough. We are most effective making an amend directly if at all possible. We'll find most people are very open to talking about amends and are glad to work on finding a way to put the past to rest. This keeps us aware of being kind to others.

When I make sincere and honest apology for a wrong I've done, I feel better for having done "the right thing."

TENTH STEP PRAYER

I pray I may continue:
To grow in understanding and effectiveness;
To take daily spot check inventories of myself;
To correct mistakes when I make them;
To take responsibility for my actions;
To be ever aware of my negative and self-defeating
   attitudes and behaviors;
To keep my willfulness in check;
To always remember I need Your help;
To keep love and tolerance of others as my code;
And to continue in daily prayer how I can best serve
   You, my Higher Power.

COMMON SENSE

We are what we think. All that we are arises with our thoughts. With our thoughts we make our world. — Buddha

Common sense is a good approach to living in our recovery program. The Tenth Step of our Program states that it is wise to pause often to analyze all our choices. Hurried remarks or actions can lead to errors. We learn that when we are wrong we promptly admit it.

That admission, of course, reflects honesty and humility at their very best. We grow in understanding and effectiveness. A hasty remark or behavior can injure or anger the person at whom it is directed. All too often, this results in embarrassment and hurt. Our responsibility to carry the message does not entitle us to "ram it down the throats" of even those who badly need our advice.

I should always think before I act or speak. Common sense reminds me, "to know what I know and to know what I don't know is knowing what it's all about."

ELEVENTH STEP PRAYER

Higher Power, as I understand You, I pray to keep my connection with You open and clear from the confusion of daily life. Through my prayers and meditations I ask especially for freedom from self-will, rationalization, and wishful thinking. I pray for the guidance of correct thought and positive action. Your will, Higher Power, not mine, be done.

CONSCIOUS CONTACT

The task ahead of us is never as great as the Power behind us. —Anonymous

Step Eleven improves our conscious contact with God. We prepare ourselves for whatever is to come when we ask only to do the will of God. The more we practice this Step, the better we get at hearing what God is telling us. Our sixth sense of intuition becomes our main sense. We begin to intuitively know what to do.

We shouldn't be surprised that we find ourselves in

service. What better task is there for us than to carry the message? Step Eleven keys us into our Power. Step Twelve exercises that Power where it can do good. It is good to practice Step Eleven before we attempt to do anything, even get out of bed in the morning.

I focus on establishing contact with and turning my will over to my Higher Power before I attempt to do anything. Step Eleven opens my ears and my heart to what I am supposed to accomplish.

TWELFTH STEP PRAYER

Dear God,

My spiritual awakening continues to unfold. The help I have received I shall pass on and give to others, both in and out of the Fellowship. For this opportunity I am grateful.

I pray most humbly to continue walking day by day on the road of spiritual progress. I pray for the inner strength and wisdom to practice the principles of this way of life in all I do and say. I need You, my friends, and the Program every hour of every day. This is a better way to live.

HELPING OTHERS

Gratitude should go forward, rather than backward. — Bill W.

When we realize how much the Program and others have helped us, it becomes our responsibility to help others. Our Twelfth Step suggests we carry the message to those who still suffer. Many of our fellows are also suffering in recovery. We need to remember to help those who may need our Fellowship as well as those in our Fellowship.

Life is no longer a dead end without hope. With the gifts we have received from the Program, we are able to help others. Our spiritual progress is easily measured by our positive actions. We are only asked to be helpful and leave the results to our Higher Power.

Bill W. said, "If you carry the message to still others, you will be making the best possible repayment for the help given you." I want to give back what I have received by sharing the Program with others.

5
CAUTION: RELAPSE TRIGGERS

The signposts to relapse are well marked. Two of the major reasons for relapse are not going to meetings and staying away from fellow members. The following are also areas to be aware of, and are the most common relapse triggers.

GLAMORIZING

We begin slipping when we begin to remember more of the good times than the bad. The program teaches us to keep our memories of the years while we were using in proper perspective. The longer we are abstinent the less we crave cocaine, but our addiction never leaves us. It is, as old timers remind us, cunning, baffling, powerful, and patient. Our addiction is waiting for us to lower our guard.

Rewriting our past is a relapse signal we watch for. When the false reality of the good times is all we remember, we are slipping into stinking thinking. Do we remember the parties, the sex, and the rush we got, or do we remember the crazy behavior that made us lose our self-esteem, lost us opportunities, or got us in trouble?

When our addiction talks to us about the drug-induced "good times," we need to remember the rest of the story and stay close to our program.

MISTAKES

We can feel a lot of unhappiness, anger, and resentment if we dwell on our past mistakes and failures. The program, our fellow members, and our Higher Power can help us in many ways, but we can't be forced to accept our own past. If we prefer to walk around with a load of shame and guilt, that's our choice.

Many people have relapsed because they couldn't let go and accept their past mistakes. The Steps and many tools can help, but as the slogan goes, "If you turn it over and don't let go of it, you'll be upside down." None of us were born perfect; we were born human. It's not surprising that this humanness, along with out-of-control drug use, has caused us trouble in our lives.

SLIPPERY PLACES AND PEOPLE

Many of us had to learn the hard way, but the advice to stay away from slippery places and people cannot be ignored. As they say in the program, "If you sit in the barber chair long enough, you're bound to get your hair cut." We have found that staying around the people and places from our using days causes many relapses.

When our ego tells us we can handle slippery places and people, "no problem," we need to talk to others in the program. For over 50 years, the Big Book of Alcoholics Anonymous has suggested that A.A. members only go to places where alcohol is served "if they have a good reason." We have never been the best judge of what is good for us. If you "have a good reason" to go where your drug of choice may be, take another 12 Step member with you.

We just had two cases in our counseling practice. A young man had to go pick up some items he had left at his dealer's house. He went with three other members, took care of business, and got out of there. A young woman in early recovery missed going to the night club for dancing. She took her sponsor and a few girlfriends from the program, and had a good time.

Holidays, vacations, concerts, special occasions can still be enjoyed, even if our drug or drugs of choice may be around, but **only** when we also take our program with us. When we take along fellow members, we take the program.

Stay away from the things that trigger our addictive thinking: pipes, needles, mirrors, etc. Stay away from situations, places, and people who may tell us "we can handle it," "one won't hurt," "it's O.K. to take a shortcut to happiness." Remember the tricks our minds play on us. We have a disease that always tells us we don't have it.

IDENTIFY, DON'T COMPARE

A stumbling block in recovery is comparing our personal program and using history with fellow members instead of identifying with them. The stories we hear in meetings often shock us. It seems hard to believe that some members could have harmed themselves so badly. We hear about arrests, bankruptcies, loss of family and home, lost jobs, abuse, violence, jail, physical injury—the list goes on. Many of us have said to ourselves, "I never was that bad. Maybe I don't really belong here."

Our sponsor and fellow members quickly straightened us out. We were comparing our histories with other members. We were told to identify with the stories, not compare. Some of us were lucky worse things hadn't happened to us while we were using. We were reminded those things hadn't happened to us "**yet.**" If we relapse, the "yets" are waiting.

PROBLEMS HAPPEN

Problems happen whether we are in recovery or not. Recovery doesn't guarantee us a life free from struggle, pain, or problems. Working the Steps strengthens us to meet crises head on. Above all, the Steps show us we never need to fear problems as we did in the old days. We learn to face problems with confidence and faith in our ability to cope. When problems bring us up against something which is a complete surprise, we meet it with an effort to do the best we can.

Problems come in all sizes. They can be minor annoyances or earthshaking adventures, but we know we always need to confront a problem as soon as it happens. There are no benefits in procrastination. Recovery doesn't promise us a life without problems, but a way to deal with them. Helping others in trouble and giving away the knowledge we've been given by coping and working through our problems helps us grow spiritually. We ask for help with problems that threaten our abstinence. We are reminded, "A problem shared is a problem halved."

STRESS

We have learned to be ever mindful of stress. We can't do everything. One of our common goals in recovery is balance: a feeling and sense of being centered. If we lean too far in one direction, we lose our balance and fall over. We can't please everyone. We can't be everything to everybody. We can't sponsor everyone, be at every meeting, or volunteer for every service opportunity. Recovery is not a race to see who can do the most.

There is a balance the program teaches us between being selfish and being everybody's "doormat." We are careful to organize our time and set priorities. We learn and practice the art of saying no. We have the right to refuse requests, to slow down and take time out, to take care of ourselves. We get too stressed out if we are not careful in organizing our time. When we're trying to do too much, we all too often remember the chemicals we used to pick ourselves up and make us mellow.

TOTAL ABSTINENCE

All 12 Step Fellowships believe in total abstinence. We don't join a 12 Step program to help us with one specific drug. When we abstain from cocaine, we abstain from all mood-changers. No, we aren't doing better switching drugs. No, we can't stay off cocaine and drink beer. No, we can't chip with a little smoke of pot.

DREAMS

It is very common to have "drunk dreams" in recovery, especially during the first year. Our minds are active while we are sleeping and dreams are a natural part. We can have dreams of using so real we feel as if we've had a relapse.

Some of these dreams can be scary. Not to worry. Our minds need time to heal. Dreaming about using won't in itself make us relapse. This is why we keep our fellow members' phone numbers handy. A late-night call to a friend or our sponsor is a great way to get back to reality.

IMMATURITY

Childish egos and immature attitudes followed many of us into recovery. It is difficult to give up our child-like need to control or our desire that all our needs be instantly met. An attitude of *I want what I want when I want it*, and desires for power, constant attention, approval, and instant pleasure have no place in recovery.

When we act like King or Queen Baby, we become impatient and frustrated. We think things aren't happening fast enough. We get into arguments because we always need to be right. We think and act like we are the center of the world. We believe that status, fame, money, and beauty are the most important things in life. When we hang on to the idea that being rebels, outlaws, and *living on the edge* is cool, we stay stuck.

The program teaches us to be other-centered, not self-centered. We care about and are interested in other people. We quit believing in Baby Power and start believing in a Higher Power.

H.A.L.T.

H.A.L.T. = Don't get too **H**ungry, or too **A**ngry, or too **L**onely, or too **T**ired. There's a lot of good advice in this simple slogan.

When we're physically weak, it affects our recovery. We learn which foods are good and bad for us, and when we're hungry, we eat.

Anger leads to resentments and can eat us up alive. In recovery, we learn how to deal with anger and cool off.

Loneliness makes us easy marks for the many voices that tempt us away from the program. We learn to get with other people, go to a meeting, or use the phone.

Fatigue makes us remember the chemical pick-me-ups we relied on before recovery. When we're tired, we need to rest.

STINKING THINKING

We learn that we don't just have a problem with addiction. We also have a thinking problem. The way we think creates our attitudes. Most relapses occur from a bad attitude. Our best thinking got us into the program.

When our thinking and attitudes are bad, we "talk the talk, but don't walk the walk." We tell people what they want to hear, but we really don't believe what we're saying. We act like big shots and don't follow the principles and disciplines of the program. Stinking thinking keeps our minds closed. We become defensive. We blame others for our problems.

We make progress and avoid relapse when we remember we are responsible for the attitudes we choose. We keep our expectations equal to the effort we put out.

COMPLACENCY

One of the biggest hazards we face is overconfidence, the idea that "I've got it made." This is complacency, an enemy of recovery. When we feel good and have the heat off us, we may begin to neglect the program. Many relapses can occur as a complete surprise when we're feeling good. We learn to think of recovery not just as reaching one goal and stopping, but as an ongoing process of making progress.

BOREDOM

When we're bored, we're saying: "O.K., Life, you're not doing your job of keeping me entertained." Boredom is a form of self-centeredness and self-pity. The attitude that those around us or the world itself is here to keep us amused is asking for trouble. That kind of thinking can screw up our attitude and take us back to the point where our addiction seems to be the only way out of boredom.

SEX

Many of us come into recovery full of shame and guilt over the crazy sex we took part in when we were under the influence. Some learned that offering drugs could get them sex. Others traded sex for drugs. Many newcomers to the program have never had sex without alcohol or drugs. Problems with sex, sexuality, sexual preference, or the negative feelings we have over our past need not send us into relapse.

The program helps us with these issues. The wisdom in A.A.'s *Big Book* is a good starting point:

> Our sex powers were God-given and therefore good, neither to be used lightly or selfishly nor to be despised and loathed.

We learn about forgiveness and respect. We learn how to become friends with others and not treat people as objects of our selfish desires.

6
PERSONAL SHARING

We would like to share with you some of the personal experiences of fellow 12 Step members.

MONEY
Stephen C. (3 years)

I've been in C.A. for a few years now and am much happier. I've had my ups and downs during recovery, but nothing has been worse than the days before the program. It seems as if it took me forever to finally accept my powerlessness over cocaine, to break down my denial. My denial was just layers and layers of shame of what I put myself through so I could get high.

I used and conned everyone to get the money for my drugs. I stole from my employer and justified it in my mind as making up for low wages. I really didn't care, though—getting high was more important.

I have made amends to the people I used. I found out I didn't need to make amends to those who were still using drugs. For one thing, they wouldn't understand. For another, I've been very careful to stay away from slippery people.

The program has taught me the real value of money. I have come to terms with the fact I pissed away thousands of dollars on cocaine. It was a very expensive education, and one I don't have to repeat if I stay close to the program.

Buying things can't make me happy. The happiness I've found in recovery doesn't come from buying it with money, but from working for it.

ACCEPTING MYSELF
Monica D. (1 year)

It took me such a long time to accept myself, and all the things I had been a part of. To find a place to put some of those memories was very difficult, because they were so painful at first. Just the very thought of some of them would wind my stomach up in a real knot of self-loathing and distrust.

Today, with a little bit of clean time under my belt, I can see those experiences for what they were. They were the stepping stones necessary for me to take to find my way to the doors of the fellowship.

Without some of those awful things happening to me, I never would have been desperate enough to change. I'm ever grateful to the program for loving me in spite of myself, and for teaching me to love myself.

TRYING TO FIGURE IT OUT
Pat L. (4 years)

For years before coming to the program, I knew that I was an addict. Instead of searching for what could be done about it, I spent long, crazy nights trying to figure out why I used. I figured that if I knew what caused me to do drugs, I could change and my using would stop. I thought deeply about my family and job—yes, even my defects of character. It never did any good. It just helped the coke make my head spin.

Then I found the program, and after a terrible period of struggling with it and myself, I stopped using. But I still managed to settled back into my familiar routine. Clean and sober now, I was still obsessed with the cause of my problems, past and present. So were many other newcomers. We all psychoanalyzed ourselves. Either our problem was that we were insecure, or else it was that we were too confident. It was a fascinating exercise, but it added nothing to our recovery.

The path to recovery, happiness, and mental health is through practicing the 12 Steps and helping others, not through self-analysis and journeys into our subconscious. It is important to know what our defects of character are (Steps Four and Ten), but to dwell on what causes us to be either crazy on drugs or miserably sober is useless.

Ours is a program of action, not of research and psychoanalysis. The wisdom of the program says quite simply that "self-knowledge availed us nothing." Our program is one of acting out a better life, of moving on to learn constructive ways of thinking and living.

DENIAL ISN'T A RIVER IN AFRICA
Bill O. (1-1/2 years)

Brother, if there was a word they threw around in treatment more than any other, "denial" takes the cake. They said it so many times and applied it to so many things, it lost all meaning for me. "You're in denial. You minimize. You've got denial. It's self-deception. It's the first reaction to loss. It's rationalizing. It's a defense tactic. It's a merry-go-round. It's intellectualizing. It's a dry drunk. It's a warning signal. It's blaming." Then there's family system denial, on and on. I do know this: the only thing denial isn't is a river in Africa.

In treatment we were shown movies on denial and assigned pamphlets to read on denial. Then we were told how to deal with denial and check all the lists in the denial pamphlets. I barely made it through the "process of dealing with denial." Yes, I denied the fact I was an addict. They say, "We're always the last to know we're an addict, because it's the only disease that tells us we're okay." I guess I also had some of the characteristics of denial. It wasn't until I was out of treatment, had a sponsor, and was attending meetings for a few months that I realized a very simple fact. The opposite of denial is acceptance. Now that is something I can understand. And there is no better way, in this recovering addict's experience, of learning about acceptance than our 12 Step program.

PROCRASTINATION
Lisa M. (6 years)

"I'll do it tomorrow" is a habit that leaves you always behind schedule. If yesterday's work is only getting done today, then how can today's work get done? It has, of course, to wait until tomorrow. Can you catch up? No. You are in the habit of procrastination. You have a black cloud over your head, made up of guilt, anxiety, worry. A feeling of failure creeps in.

Our program suggests living "One Day At A Time." We try to do today's work today. What if we put off the first step of the work? No job, even school, office, or career will give us satisfaction unless we see the value of our day's work. Satisfaction comes from doing the job on time, reaching our goal "just for today." If procrastination had an effect only on oneself, it wouldn't be so bad. But no, it puts a strain on everyone around us. Tight schedules leave little time for conversation or for relaxed meal times, and no time to fit into the family activities. Procrastination tends to lock you out of your community—even the community of our Fellowship. How can you share when you're in a state of mind which is preoccupied with yourself and your problems?

Breaking the habit will allow you to participate in home life and the program. The ability to concentrate, to use your time well, is everything. It is self-control. It's the program in action. The Fourth Step speaks of instincts gone wild. We must get control of our instincts.

When you're tired, you have feelings of uneasiness. These feelings come from stress, and the strain of always rushing around. Uneasiness also comes from an undernourished spirit, one that never has time to go away to a quiet place and rest awhile. The Eleventh Step seeks the will of God. Haven't we enough to deal with in today's troubles without making a double load for tomorrow?

Benjamin Franklin said, "Do you love life? Then do not squander time, for that is the stuff life is made of." The 12 Steps are the same for everyone. We are all given the choice and the means to break the habit of procrastination, so that we may be free to strive for spiritual growth in our lives.

AS WE UNDERSTOOD
Billie Jo A. (3 years)

Step Three is the big one. Taking this Step is often the key to whether or not we stay clean. I am positive it is the only road to spiritual progress.

Before the program, after being "failed" by others over and over again, I relied solely on my own resources. My motto was, "If you want something done, do it yourself." So when it was suggested that I make a decision to turn my will and my life over to the care of God, I hesitated at first, feeling scared and confused.

Could a Higher Power be trusted to care for me? I wondered. It seemed that no one else in my life had ever cared. How could I trust anyone or anything? Hadn't I been raped, beaten up, and abused? My experience did not lead me to believe I could ever safely trust anyone. God was a force I turned to as a child each night in prayer, but I later came to think God had no power over the dark side of human behavior, and thus no power to keep me safe from heartache. Early on, I had given up hope of a Higher Power. I thought self-will was the answer to living.

Recently, after eighteen months of living clean and sober, I started feeling this way again. I said to myself, "Maybe the only way I will become productive is by pulling myself up by my own bootstraps." Life's daily stresses and living near poverty level became too much for me. Doubt about the existence of God crept into my mind. How could God care for me and yet leave me to my own devices? I had done the footwork, so where were the results? Was the program just another con game?

It became clear to me that I was in a spiritual crisis.

Although I felt myself slipping into despair and self-pity, I continued to pray. "Get to a meeting" was the message received.

Only after deep prayer did the memories of the miracle hit me. I'm clean! I see others getting and staying clean after years of active addiction. My heart is full and my mind is clear! I do have enough today. God **does** care for me—one day at a time.

When darkness seems to be closing in on every side, I can take comfort knowing that as long as I continue to make a daily decision to turn my will and life over to a caring God, my daily needs will be met. Perhaps things do not come together quite the way I think they should. I may not be able to feel my Higher Power working in my life. Everything may be falling apart around me. Despair and discouragement may engulf me. Yet deep in my soul my Third Step decision will build a spiritual fortress for me where I can take refuge.

DATING
Dan F. (2 years)

I was quite shocked in early recovery to realize I didn't know the first thing about dating. I had gone out with a lot of women when I was using. As long as I had coke, I was remarkably popular. To ask someone out, I just asked if she would like to do some coke. Getting a date was easy, and they all said I was the best, and they all said they loved me (as long as the coke lasted).

I didn't think much about dating in early recovery. I was just hanging on and going to a lot of meetings. The thought of someone going out with me just because I was me was confusing. Why would anyone want to go with me without some "hook," money or drugs?

My sponsor suggested I first learn how to be friends with women before I began dating. It took awhile to get my head on straight about this area of my recovery. Recovery means more than just stopping drugs. It has to do with every aspect of the way you treat yourself and others.

THE SLIP
Nancy P. (2-1/2 years)

I had been in the program three months when I had a slip. As I look back on it now, it's easy to explain what happened. I had stopped using and joined the program just to get my boss off my back.

It was easy to go back out and find coke to do. I knew exactly where to go. The day after my slip I was overwhelmed by guilt and very disappointed with myself. Somehow I got the courage to go back to my group and tell them about my slip. I'm glad I didn't stay out there on a long slip before I went back. My group told me I hadn't lost everything; I had just made a mistake, nothing more and nothing less.

I look back now, two years later, and think of my slip as an educational experience. I started to listen and work the program when I went back. I began to change my behavior so further slips wouldn't happen. But this time I did it for myself, not for anyone else.

GRATITUDE
Mary S. (5 years)

My biggest sense of gratitude, probably, comes from my having been granted an increasing awareness of my self-destructive half. I've learned to accept my addiction as a prime trigger for this self-destruction. I've been given twelve channels to explore myself mentally, physically, spiritually, and emotionally in conjunction with everything else.

If it hadn't been for my defects of character, I doubt I could have sustained my abuse of drugs. The program teaches me to recognize my defects. This knowledge is so important in preventing me from repeating disasters from which I never learned.

This is gratitude born from self-examination, based on the observations of clean and sober people. I feel further gratitude for being in recovery now, and for the fine vision of the future with its concepts of humility, Higher Power, simplicity, reality, and trust.

I am learning to regard life as a loan which, like all loans, is to be repaid. As a custodian, I must treat life with care. Also, within the limits of my understanding and ability, I believe I must apply the right and seek the good, shun fear and seek faith. With my fellow man I should look for love, dignity, and humility. At my end, I hope to feel fulfillment and gratitude for the loan rather than malice, hate, fear, or failure.

I feel great beauty around me. I hope these thoughts convey it. My effort has been well rewarded, and I am grateful.

WILLING TO CHANGE
Diana M. (2-1/2 years)

At a very young age, I recognized what I believed to be my "difference." I didn't have steady friends; I spent lots of time alone, and I believed I was smarter than most kids. I didn't know it at the time, but I was lonely.

I was first introduced to liquor as a curative for female cramps when I complained to my parents of pain. I believe a seed was planted to numb the pain of whatever hurt me.

I started on drugs in the late sixties, acid, reefer, pills, cheap wine . . . I usually abused whatever substance the man in my life abused. I thought it brought us together on a higher plane; I thought it made our relationship "spiritual." I thought sex was better. I suppose, in fact, everything was just more intense. The intensity blocked reality.

In the winter of 1985 my job announced that in thirty days it would begin conducting random urine tests. I panicked. I asked my boyfriend, "If I can't get high, what now?" He explained that cocaine leaves the body in only 72 hours. I had never done cocaine but I knew exactly what to do with it. I snorted a few lines, complained about the cost, and went to bed.

A few days later he brought home a pipe. From the first hit I was hooked. I tried to be cool and put on a good appearance. I would suggest saving some for later or tomorrow, but I knew he wouldn't stop so it was safe to suggest it. I understood almost immediately that cocaine was addictive, but I did not understand that I was an addict. I smoked for six months. Then one day I realized that cocaine was the most important thing in my life and I stopped. I had stopped and started with other drugs and liquor for years. Stopping coke should be easy. But it wasn't. My boyfriend continued to use, and when I forbade drugs in the house he seldom came home.

For four months I didn't use drugs or alcohol, and then he asked for help. Through A.A. we were referred to a C.A. meeting. I admitted to the fellowship I was an addict. I knew from the comments in that room that I was one among many and that I didn't have to be alone any more.

My boyfriend and I continued to go to that one meeting a week. Eventually I went alone. When I realized that the meetings weren't helping him and he was going to continue to use, I stopped going. I continued to stay clean, but I was suffering more spiritually and emotionally than I had in all the years I used and drank. Finally he moved out. I had been clean for a year, and had wanted cocaine every day of that year.

I don't know why but one day when I was feeling like I wanted to die because of the deep hole inside of me, I called a woman in the program, whining about how miserable I was. She asked me if I was praying (no), going to meetings (no), or talking to people on the program (no). Because I was in such pain, I was now ready to go to any lengths to feel better. I began going to five or six meetings a week. I took phone numbers and eventually I was able to call people; I began praying, and I got a sponsor.

At first it seemed like nothing was changing, but, in fact, much did. Though I'm not aware of when it happened, the compulsion to use left, but the pain did not.

Then one day, I was praying and I realized that though my faith was actually quite minute, I did believe I was praying to God as I understood Him. With this new strength I was able to let go of my boyfriend. Our relationship had been the source of much pain, and for the first time, I was able to say to myself and to God "I don't want this kind of pain any more."

At my sponsor's suggestion I got involved in service work. I began to care about people other than me. Though I am still self-centered I know I am not the same person I was when I stopped using.

My faith is stronger than ever, and each morning I ask God to keep me sober. I also make a decision that I will be happy. Though problems arise, people hurt my feelings, and I act on my defects, I now reflect on the situation immediately. I don't always admit when I've been wrong, but I always make a decision not to let anyone or anything change the way I feel about life, and that is: grateful to be alive clean and sober.[3]

CHANGES
E.G. (2-1/2 YEARS)

I'm an addict and an alcoholic. I'm also a miracle. A miracle because I didn't wake up with an overpowering obsession to get loaded and because I am changing. That's what it is all about to me—change, whether it's my reactions, my thoughts, my behavior, or a change in my beliefs. The longer I am clean, the more I see that cocaine was a symptom. I've done heroin, LSD, downers, alcohol, and other drugs, but cocaine whipped and humbled me. From using in affluent places to waiting for more on street corners, that was my journey.

Now I'm on a journey of another kind. It is the journey through the Steps of this program. I came from a family that was emotionally incapable of showing affection or sharing feelings. I was always discouraged and felt guilty whenever I had desires or feelings because I was unable to express them. Consequently I was a very angry child. I can share my war stories of how it was, but I know today that what matters is how I was.

Progress in sobriety not perfection. Some days "Don't drink or use no matter what" is all I can manage. I have been clean and sober for over two years now after many years of resistance to the Fellowship. I know now that when I hear and feel the similarities instead of the differences I have a better chance at this way of life.

Before, I only understood street corners, the hustle, manipulation, and images. But when I came to the Fellowship, it showed me hope, solutions, truth, and love. I don't always think on these terms today, but I realize that I don't have to be directed by my past thoughts and actions. The secret past is no longer a secret. My past is no longer my Higher Power.

Someone once told me that Steps One, Two, and Three are learning to turn it over. Steps Four through Nine are what we turn over, and Steps Ten through Twelve are how we keep it turned over.

Today I believe in what the Big Book says about the root of my disease being self-centered, selfish fear. Today the answer when I feel fear or when I have a self-created dilemma is either to treat it chemically or treat it spiritually. I thank Cocaine Anonymous for being a channel of hope for me today. There is a way to live with feelings and thoughts without using drugs or alcohol.

One other thing that helps when I'm not feeling centered or when I experience those feelings of low self-esteem, self-pity, and fear is knowing that the best thing I can do is show up, pay attention, and tell the truth.

The reality of it is that once I started drinking or using, I was powerless—I could not stop. I spent years going in and out of this program being directed by my past and reacting to my old thoughts. Today the principles help to guide me and clear away the past. I have a better understanding of fellowship; i.e., meetings, people, recovery, the Steps, and helping others. I can take nothing and be the same, or take nothing and change. I am grateful for that choice. If you believe the same, you'll stay the same; if you believe differently, you'll change.[3]

YOUR BABY'S A JUNKIE
B.M. (1 YEAR)

Marijuana . . . Quaaludes . . . Speed . . . P.C.P. . . . Heroin . . . Cocaine . . .

How deceiving these drugs can be! This is the story of a twelve-year-old kid who thought drugs were the answer, only to find himself, years later, in a federal prison serving a twenty-year sentence without the possibility of parole for trying to be "one of the boys."

It seems that since I was a kid something was always missing in my life, something I never understood until now. I tried to fill this void with street gangs, drugs, girls, fancy clothes, big cars, and money. I never cared much for school, thinking it was "jive." I smoked my first joint at twelve years old, thinking it would make me part of something and chasing a dream that turned out to be a nightmare. Even though I swore I would never use anything heavier than marijuana, it was no more than two months later I was taking "downers" for the same reasons. As the void in my life got bigger, that need to be accepted also got stronger and so did the drugs I was taking.

Soon after this some of my friends and I robbed a candy store for forty dollars and change to buy two ounces of marijuana, which we used to start dealing nickel bags. We ran a nickel and dime business from the street corner. There were times when we had cars backed up for half a block with people trying to "cop" from us, especially on Friday nights.

I got not only money from dealing, also acceptance, prestige, girls, and a feeling of importance. It surely did feel good to be thought of as the "main man" in the neighborhood among my peers, especially at the age of thirteen.

The problem, though, was that I was trying to fill this void, which just seemed to keep getting bigger and bigger. Soon the girls and the dealing just couldn't fill it. There was no peace or satisfaction in anything for me.

When you're struggling to keep up a reputation, you have to keep up with the times. At this time, the older fellows were shooting speed. At first I said, "I'll never put a needle in my arm!" But, overcome with peer pressure and wanting to live up to my reputation, I found myself (at thirteen) taking my first shot of speed. Within seconds, as the drug went through my veins, I remember saying, "I want more."

I was aware of the old rumor that says "one hit and you're hooked." Maybe it's not true that you're physically addicted, but I tell you from the bottom of my heart that from my first I was hooked!

My friends and I swore we would only do it on weekends. That was fine, for a while, until summer.

Even though I frequently heard a little voice that I didn't understand within myself telling me that what I was doing was wrong, the feelings from the drugs were too strong to resist. I had no adults in whom I could confide or to seek counsel from or guidance. Not that my parents wouldn't have listened; I was just afraid they wouldn't understand, and I didn't want to let them down.

About half-way through my junior year at high school I was introduced to the big "H," heroin. I thought for sure that it was the answer to all my problems, and sure that it was . . . temporary. By summer I found myself going through $50 to $100 a day. Eventually I was so sick that my father called the doctor. I'll never forget the look on my father's face when the doctor told him, "Your baby's a junkie!" Even though my father was disappointed and hurt so badly that I can't find the right words to describe it, he never gave up on me. We tried drug program after drug program. Nothing we did seemed to be the answer to my problems. I put my family through pure torture.

So, to make a very long story relatively short, I began a life of dealing cocaine and living in the "fast lane." In plain words, for a while, I had everything that could be bought with money. Then one day I found myself in solitary confinement in the county jail waiting to be transferred to federal prison. I had just received a twenty-year sentence without possibility of parole. For me what was missing from my life and from my recovery was my Higher Power. I found that Higher Power in that jail cell, when I confessed my life was a mess and I needed a savior.

I suppose that if there is any advice I would give it's that drugs are not the answer to the void. You can take it from me, a kid that learned too late, but at least I learned.[3]

MOTIVATION
Tricia T. (1 year)

In spite of being an addict I am still a human being who believes she has a role to play in my life community. Over the recent year, I have built up a far more positive image of myself, which has enabled me to develop meaningful relationships with others with more confidence in my ability to do so.

Over the years I have experienced loneliness, depression, and many times a complete lack of confidence. Bad childhood experiences caused by my alcoholic father contributed to my low self-image and lack of motivation to take actions to my own advantage. I think action is the result of motivation. Acting without motivation is a losing game.

The benefits we receive from acting with motivation are increased interest, an awareness that we are making new discoveries, and a feeling of peace because we have had the courage to act.

Now with the help of the program I am thinking along more positive lines. My thinking has changed. I have come to accept myself. Perhaps more importantly, I have managed to come to terms with my bad childhood memories. Now I live in the present and look forward to a better future with the program and my fellow members.

LETTING GO
Donna T. (6 years)

Six years ago I had to let go. My life was unmanageable and I was a mess. I had to let go of my family and let them get along without me so I could get into recovery. If I hadn't, I would be dead now and my children would be living with terrible emotional scars, even worse than the ones they carry now.

First I had to let go of the idea that the survival of my two kids depended on my managing their lives. Then I had to let go of guilt born of old ideas such as, "A **good** person doesn't leave her family and take care of herself. A mother always takes care of her family and puts herself last." And on and on.

I wrenched myself away from them and entered a treatment facility. They got along just fine without me. I got myself back into the world of reality, ever-increasing sanity, and peace of mind by applying myself to the program with my full energy and time, without distractions and demands of family members. My Higher Power took care of me and my family.

Today my children are back with me. They chose to re-enter my life. I left that up to them. I had found I could not handle even my own life—how could I manage theirs? By letting go, I let my Higher Power give us the direction, protection, and affection we needed. Many people have been placed in our lives. I am very grateful for my six years of recovery.

To let go is to fear less and love more. To let go doesn't mean we stop caring. To let go is to admit powerlessness. Letting go of my old ideas has freed me to make progress. Every single idea that has been discarded has returned with better things over and over. And I believe the best is yet to come.

NO MORE RUNNING AWAY
JAY E. (1-1/2 YEARS)

I was a possible drug addict in my early teens, because of the many experiences which took place in my life. When I was faced with problems I couldn't handle, I ran away from them. I turned my back on reality, refusing to accept any unpleasant situation. I ran away from everything life stood for. I would never ask for help or seek out guidance. I knew it all! So I always took the easy way out.

In high school I found the ultimate escape from reality—stay high on drugs and alcohol. I found escape not only from dealing with problems, but from life itself. I spent my time hanging around with others who were doing the same thing.

I dropped out of high school as my drug reality took over my whole life. Self-pity threw me into despair. I found myself in a hell of my own making. Everyone rejected me. Friends and family stayed away from me. The only reality that was comfortable was that of drugs. I wanted desperately to get out. I looked for the end.

A drunk driving ticket got me the help that turned me around. I was so angry about being found out, but I chose to go into treatment instead of jail. After the second week in treatment listening to others and seeing some films, I asked for help. I found it.

I've finally walked out of the valley of fear, anger, and confusion. My rebellion against everyone and everything is part of my past. The program has given me the way to put my broken life back together. I've become a part of what I used to turn my back on.

FEELINGS
Deb D. (3 years)

Oh, for release from the pain of growing up! Unfortunately, the only way to have permanent release from this pain is to complete the process on a daily basis, and start it again the next day.

"At times I feel like screaming, crying, or smashing something." Feelings like this were part of my old way of life. The only way I coped with them was to wipe them out with drugs and a big phony front. Today they're not such a great part of my life any more. They do still exist for me, though, and every day I try to use the Twelve Steps to come to terms with them.

Why do I feel this way? Frustration, self-pity, too-high expectations of myself and others, self-doubt, feelings of inferiority, confusion—I still feel these emotions at times, even though through the last few years of recovery I've learned most of these are unrealistic, negative, and useless.

Some people would have me believe (myself included at times) that I shouldn't be feeling like this so far into my recovery. To this I say nonsense! The program has taught me there is no set time limit for recovery from drug addiction. I may never fully recover from the personality disorders I suffer at times.

I am at present involved in another spiritual spring-cleaning. I'm convinced that the Steps and my fellow members will put me in touch with the key to my particular hang-ups.

Sometimes, being the fallible human I am, I allow situations, instead of my Higher Power, to take control of my life. When that happens, it's hard to get out from under the pile of garbage I've taken on.

The way I feel about being alive and sober **never** changes. Even with all the hassles I create, on top of those that really exist, I still love life clean and sober. But please forgive my humanity and super-sensitivity—sometimes I hurt inside and don't see what to do about it. At least I know now that the knowledge and experience are there for me to tap into, if I only will.

I know, if I keep making progress, that time, faith, and the love of my fellow human beings will let me grow the way I am meant to grow.

NEVER TOO YOUNG TO DIE
S.F. (10 MONTHS)

I'm a very grateful recovering addict. My story probably doesn't differ much from anyone else's but I feel the need to share some of my experience, strength, and hope to encourage others.

I believe I was an addict before I ever picked up drugs, because I never fit in anywhere, though I certainly tried. I'd pretend to be a biker, or a hippie, or a flower child. Wherever I was, I changed to be like the people I was with, all the time feeling like I had to prove myself.

I never felt loved or wanted. I tried to make people love me. I would make people write "I love you" down on a piece of paper and keep it in my wallet as "proof." I felt so unloved. I'd do insane things for attention. Once I slit my wrists in school. I didn't want to die, I just wanted to hurt myself bad enough so someone would come visit me in the hospital and pay some attention to me.

It felt like I fought for year for love and affection. After so long, I gave up. I took the attitude that I don't need anyone. I could do everything on my own and didn't want anyone to be around me. I didn't need you. I acted like nothing bothered me. I could handle everything. No one was going to get the best of me ever again.

Little did I know drugs eased that pain. Pretty soon there weren't enough drugs in the world to ease all the pain and rejection I felt. I had to stay numb twenty-four hours a day, seven days a week. I hated myself, I had no self-worth, self-respect or self-esteem. I allowed people to treat me like dirt, because I figured it was better than having no one at all.

I moved out of my dad's home when I was fifteen. I was determined to be "free." I didn't realize I was already in prison. I locked myself in a world of games and lies with fake people and false places. I always talked about all the places I'd go and all the things I'd do, but I always wound up in the same place doing the same thing, getting high. I was all talk.

I moved from place to place, always running, always trying to find happiness.

Using progressed—I stole and lied so much I began to believe my own lies. I was a "professional" when it came to making people feel sorry for me.

When I turned seventeen, I had a $300-a-day habit. I couldn't smoke enough coke, or anything else for that matter. I got into a car accident and then started having convulsions.

I've been to three treatment programs and I learned I'd never get help until I helped myself. I changed a lot since then. I used to think I was too young to die, too young to have a problem. Hogwash.

I surrendered and became willing to do anything it took. I have a great sponsor today, more friends that truly love me than I ever imagined. I work the Steps to the best of my ability. I have happiness in my life. No more clinging to my old image—I've found self-respect, self-worth, and (a little more) self-esteem.

I hold my head up high today because I'm worth something. I love myself. I speak at jails and treatment centers. I sponsor two women, and I'm involved in service work. It's so great to truly be free. I have real fun today, dancing and going to conventions.

I'm truly a miracle. I've never been so happy in my life. In four days I'll be nineteen, and in two more months I'll be celebrating my first year. I know I have a life-and-death disease. This is no game. I have a real patient monkey on my back waiting to kill me. But I choose life today.

Please don't ever give up on anyone. I was the one they said would never make it. But because you people loved me when I could not love myself, and you people didn't give up on me when I gave up on myself, I live today.

I could never thank you all enough for your help. I owe Narcotics Anonymous everything. I will be forever in debt to this program. Than you, N.A., for my life.

I *am* too young to die.[4]

7
THE PROMISES

On page 83 of the Big Book of Alcoholics Anonymous, there begins a long paragraph worthy of study. The sentences in that paragraph have been referred to as "The Promises."

We who are finding spiritual growth should frequently take time to examine the promises we find in working our program. We always discover that we are working toward a definite purpose for promised rewards.

Just before the listing of the Promises, we read that we will be surprised at the spiritual progress we have made after finishing the Ninth Step. The Ninth Step concerns making direct amends.

We once believed that we needed a certain substance or behavior in order to avoid loneliness and boredom. The Promises get rid of that idea. We are made aware that "God wants us to be happy, joyous, and free."

After completing the journey through the first Nine Steps, the Promises begin to unfold for us.

THE FIRST PROMISE

We will know a new freedom and happiness. —*Big Book*

A new freedom and happiness for us is an almost unbelievable Promise. Before recovery, we had little choice and less freedom. Everything we did had to be set up to meet the demands of our compulsion. Try as hard as we possibly could, we could never prevent the consuming urge of our addiction. A powerful compulsion took over all our waking hours.

Our lives were controlled by our desires. There was a constant need to bow to the demands of our addiction. It made all our decisions for us. There was no freedom and only a small bit of happiness at the very best. We always had to "pay the piper," and we knew it. We were slaves, like it or not. When freedom came with abstinence, so came joy, gratitude, and love for others and ourselves.

We once believed we could control our addiction. When we found it wasn't possible, we felt deep depression, guilt, shame, and remorse. We felt we no longer had freedom. Recovery finally gave us a choice. Promises do come true.

THE SECOND PROMISE

We will not regret the past nor wish to shut the door upon it. —Big Book

In the program, we begin to "clean house" and "get our acts together." As long as we denied and tried to hide from the world, and ourselves, the truth of what kind of person we were when we were using, there would be no approach to abstinence and little possibility of ever preventing relapse.

Without awareness of what the past did to us, we, even if clean and sober, will find ourselves unable to truly carry the message of hope and the gift of a new life to those who desperately need it. Relating our past experiences builds a common ground of love and service between us and the ones for whose awakening we have declared ourselves responsible. Because of that honesty, newcomers can come to realize that they are not alone and that they too can "make it."

THE THIRD PROMISE

We will comprehend the word serenity and know peace. —Big Book

When we read this Promise, we nod our heads eagerly. When we first decided to shake the bondage of addiction through the love, encouragement, deep concern, and help from newfound friends, we knew what serenity felt like. A life of serenity and security comes naturally when we realize that all those who preceded us in our Fellowship have not only had the same problems, but have found solutions which they willingly pass on to us.

Peace of mind is new to us. Serenity becomes refreshing and comfortable as we realize we are free men and women and come to admit to ourselves that we have experienced a miracle.

With that awareness, we find true belief. With abstinence comes mental clarity. Serenity gives us a perfect climate in which spiritual progress can grow.

THE FOURTH PROMISE

No matter how far down the scale we have gone, we will see how our experience can benefit others. —Big Book

What excitement comes to us when we discover that we are not useless human beings! When we drank or used, we thought we were doomed to be incompetent, unworthy, and useless persons. No more!

Our escape from the depths of despair makes us feel needed and trusted. Others listen to our stories of how we were, what happened, and what we are today. They cry out, "That's me. I was that way. I did all those same things."

We come to know we deserve that trust, that companionship, that acceptance. We are worthy human beings. We can help others experience miracles. When we tell of our degrading existence with alcohol and drugs, we are useful and important to those who listen. Our negative experiences become positive forces in helping others find the road to recovery.

Recovery brings us the realization that we can become helpful people by sharing those very experiences that made us feel worthless.

THE FIFTH PROMISE

The feeling of uselessness and self-pity will disappear. —Big Book

When we were deep within the bewilderment and agony of our addiction, we often moaned, "What's the use? Nobody cares." We considered ourselves "lost people." We thought we were incapable of ever doing anything worthwhile for anyone, including ourselves. Shame and guilt made us wallow in self-pity, but we never blamed ourselves. It was always those people, places, and things out there that made us victims.

We complained, "They did it to me. I'm not to blame. If it hadn't been for bad luck .... I was just in the wrong place at the wrong time."

In recovery, we often refer to self-pity as the PLOMs ("poor little old me"). We learn to recognize and avoid the PLOMs by working our program and by focusing on positive things.

When we surrendered to our addiction, we were always sure we had been betrayed by others. We were sorry for ourselves. Now the promise has come true. We are useful and free of self-pity.

THE SIXTH PROMISE

We shall lose interest in selfish things and gain interest in our fellows. —Big Book

We came into the program as experts in dishonesty, deceit, envy, and self-pity. Selfishness was an emotion that fitted us well. We were shameless in the ways we found useful in taking advantage of other people. The victims of our selfishness most often were those who loved us and tried to help us.

Our self-importance was based on unreality and was the effect of addicted behavior. We engaged in far out thinking that reached the heights of fantasy. Our selfishness and self-centeredness developed within all of us a sick ego that turned into a powerhouse of grandiosity. The arrogance of an ego-driven addict was a drawback to willingness. In such a state of being, only miracles could help us.

In our addiction, our selfishness made us "me first" people. In recovery, we are interested in the well-being of others. This has caused our self-interest to disappear.

THE SEVENTH PROMISE

Self-seeking will slip away. —Big Book

When we were using, constant self-seeking was our whole existence. Being forced to cut down or stop was impossible to imagine. It was an invasion of our right to live as we wished. It didn't matter that that choice was creating physical suffering and mental anguish for us and those who loved us.

We were always on the defensive. Our answer to any accusation or plea to quit was always "it's none of your business," or "let me live my own life."

With abstinence, we began to practice understanding, humility, gratitude, caring and sharing with others, openmindedness, faith in our program's recovery Steps, love of others, and belonging in a world of positiveness and action. We are beginning to attain a life where we realize we are truly people who need people.

When we became abstinent, we learned that making constant spiritual progress is what life is truly all about, and the self-seeking slipped away.

THE EIGHTH PROMISE

Our whole attitude and outlook on life will change.
—Big Book

Before the program, the only changes in our lives were in the substances we were using, our companions, or the places we went to use. We only changed the way we obeyed the commands of our compulsion. What didn't change was the fact that our lives always became worse.

We never admitted that our addiction was our enemy. We always considered it to be a friend in times of need. We believed it was the only way to enjoy life until it began to destroy that life. Then we realized it must be put entirely out of our lives if we were to survive.

Our attitudes and outlook on life changed for the better in every way when we began to practice abstinence and work the Steps.

Today we see exciting changes occurring physically, emotionally, and spiritually. We are no longer slaves to the limited changes dictated by our addiction.

THE NINTH PROMISE

Fear of people and of economic insecurity will leave us. —Big Book

When we were deep in our compulsions and obsessions, we were afraid of people, especially those who loved us. We were terrified we would not have the necessities of life. And we usually lost both.

Addiction so warped our minds, we were constantly fantasizing dangers from sources we could not identify or bring into focus. These fantasies became our reality. All the "ghosts that never were" could be traced to one major fear: that of the unknown. We distrusted people, places, and things.

Now we welcome them. Our new friends, surroundings, and tools for living are life-saving. Now when "fear knocks, faith answers – and no one is there." Our program teaches us to trust ourselves, others, and our Higher Power. The rest takes care of itself.

The only things we used to trust were those we were addicted to. When we began to put our trust in the program and our Higher Power, the destruction stopped and the recovery began.

THE TENTH PROMISE

We will instinctively know how to handle situations which used to baffle us. —Big Book

By using such slogans as "Easy Does It," "One Day at a Time," or "Together We Can Do What I Can't," we find solutions for problems that seemed unsolvable before. By working the Steps, we learn to face up to and solve the problems of everyday living that used to cause us to seek relief in our addictions.

We no longer have doubts about our ability to do for ourselves what we once expected others to do for us. If we don't know the answers, we know we can find them by asking the advice of fellow members who have faced the same problems.

The instincts which once compelled us toward our addiction have been redirected toward solving problems during recovery. We are confident that there are solutions to all problems, including some we haven't faced yet. We no longer have to dodge what we used to feel were certain failures.

We use the tools built by those who have already experienced the problems we are facing for the first time.

THE ELEVENTH PROMISE

We will suddenly realize that God is doing for us what we could not do for ourselves. —Big Book

When we are new in recovery and survive a major problem or make progress, we try to explain it by saying we have been saved by coincidence. Then our new friends are quick to tell us that there are no coincidences in recovery, only miracles. God is doing for us what we could not do for ourselves.

As we meditate on this Promise, we must practice patience, belief, and trust in our Higher Power. God always lets us know that miracles come in His time, not ours.

This Promise tells us we must accept God's help, not merely be resigned to it. We must let go of our problems personally and turn them over to God with faith.

When we used, our higher power was the substance we were using. We seldom admitted it. The Eleventh Promise tells me we have found a Higher Power that can and will do great things for us in spite of ourselves.

THE TWELFTH PROMISE

[The Promises] will always materialize if we work for them. —Big Book

Emotional growth and the fulfillment of the Promises are not gifts we receive without any effort on our part. We must earn the results by serious, dedicated work. The Steps are the tools we use to do that work.

We can think of progress as a partnership between us and our Higher Power. Directions are given and the Promises are made good to us when we follow those directions.

We must first develop complete openmindedness before we can even start to work the necessary parts of our program. We must develop an attitude of rigorous honesty. Finally, we must rid ourselves of denial, deceit, taking shortcuts, holding on to old ideas, and being satisfied with half-measures. All this must be done before we ever taste the success of the Promises made to us.

Our meditations bring us to the realization that we must always follow instructions in order to succeed in spiritual matters. God gives directions clearly. Unless we do the footwork, nothing will happen.

8
SLOGANS

1. Easy Does It
2. First Things First
3. Live And Let Live
4. But For The Grace Of God
5. Think . . . Think . . . Think
6. One Day At A Time
7. Let Go And Let God
8. K.I.S.S. = Keep It Simple Stupid
9. Act As If . . .
10. This Too Shall Pass
11. Expect A Miracle
12. I Can't . . . God Can . . . I Think I'll Let Him
13. If It Works . . . Don't Fix It
14. Keep Coming Back . . . It Works If You Work It
15. Stick With The Winners
16. Identify, Don't Compare
17. Recovery Is A Journey, Not A Destination
18. Faith Without Works Is Dead
19. You Aren't Required To Like It, You're Only Required To Do It
20. To Thine Own Self Be True
21. I Came; I Came To; I Came To Believe
22. Live In The Now

23. If God Seems Far Away, Who Moved?
24. Turn It Over
25. Utilize, Don't Analyze
26. The Elevator Is Broken, Use The Steps
27. We Are Only As Sick As Our Secrets
28. There Are No Coincidences In The Program
29. Be Part Of The Solution, Not The Problem
30. Sponsors: Have One - Use One - Be One
31. I Can't Handle It God; You Take Over
32. Keep An Open Mind
33. It Works—it Really Does!
34. Willingness Is The Key
35. More Will Be Revealed
36. You Will Intuitively Know
37. You Will Be Amazed
38. No Pain . . . No Gain
39. Go For It
40. Principles Before Personalities
41. Do It Sober
42. Let It Begin With Me
43. Just For Today
44. Sober 'N Crazy
45. Pass It On
46. It's In The Book
47. You Either Is—or You Ain't
48. Before You Say: I Can't . . . Say: I'll Try
49. Don't Quit 5 Minutes Before The Miracle Happens
50. Some Of Us Are Sicker Than Others
51. We're All Here Because We're Not All There
52. Addiction Is An Equal Opportunity Destroyer
53. Practice An Attitude Of Gratitude

54. The Road To Recovery Is A Simple Journey For Confused People With A Complicated Disease
55. Living In The Here And Now
56. God Is Never Late
57. Have A Good Day Unless You've Made Other Plans
58. Shit Happens
59. It Takes Time
60. 90 Meetings 90 Days
61. You Are Not Alone
62. Wherever You Go, There You Are
63. Our Need Is God's Opportunity
64. Use The 24-hour Plan
65. Make Use Of Telephone Therapy
66. Stay Clean And Sober For Yourself
67. Look For Similarities Rather Than Differences
68. Live Your Life So You Will Never Have To Say "If Only"
69. Remember That Drug Addiction Is Incurable, Progressive, And Fatal
70. Try Not To Place Conditions On Your Recovery
71. When All Else Fails Follow Directions
72. Count Your Blessings
73. Share Your Happiness
74. Respect The Anonymity Of Others
75. Share Your Pain
76. Let Go Of Old Ideas
77. Try To Replace Guilt With Gratitude
78. What Goes Around, Comes Around
79. Change Is A Process, Not An Event
80. Take The Cotton Out Of Your Ears And Put It In Your Mouth

81. Call Your Sponsor Before, Not After, You Start Using
82. Sick And Tired Of Being Sick And Tired
83. Seven Days Without A Meeting Makes One Weak
84. To Keep It, You Have To Give It Away
85. Man's Extremity Is God's Opportunity
86. The Price For Serenity And Sanity Is Self-sacrifice
87. Serenity = Reality = Inner Peace And Strength
88. Take What You Can Use And Leave The Rest
89. What If . . .
90. Yeah But . . .
91. If Only . . .
92. Help Is Only A Phone Call Away
93. Around The Program Or In The Program?
94. You Can't Give Away What You Don't Have
95. On The Beam Or Off The Beam
96. Welcome And "Keep Coming Back"
97. Anger Is But One Letter Away From Danger
98. Courage To Change . . .
99. Easy Does It, But Do It
100. Bring The Body And The Mind Will Follow

Cocaine Anonymous

"Cocaine Anonymous" is a fellowship of men and women who share their experience, strength, and hope with each other that they solve their common problem, and help others to recover from addiction. The only requirement for membership is a desire to stop using cocaine and all other mind-altering substances. There are no dues or fees for membership; we are self-supporting through our own contributions. C.A. is not allied with any sect, denomination, politics, organization, or institution; does not wish to engage in any controversy; neither endorses nor opposes any causes. Our primary purpose is to stay free from cocaine and all other mind-altering substances, and to help others achieve the same freedom.

Adapted and reprinted with permission of A.A. Grapevine, Inc.

The Twelve Steps Of Cocaine Anonymous

1. We admitted we were powerless over cocaine and all other mind-altering substances—that our lives have become unmanageable.
2. Came to believe that a Power greater than ourselves could restore us to sanity.
3. Made a decision to turn our will and our lives over to the care of God *as we understood Him*.
4. Made a searching and fearless moral inventory of ourselves.
5. Admitted to God, to ourselves, and to another human being the exact nature of our wrongs.
6. Were entirely ready to have God remove all these defects of character.
7. Humbly asked Him to remove our shortcomings.
8. Made a list of all persons we had harmed, and became willing to make amends to them all.
9. Made direct amends to such people wherever possible, except when to do so would injure them or others.
10. Continued to take personal inventory and when we were wrong promptly admitted it.
11. Sought through prayer and meditation to improve our conscious contact with God *as we understood Him*, praying only for knowledge of His will for us and the power to carry that out.
12. Having had a spiritual awakening as the result of these steps, we tried to carry this message to addicts, and to practice these principles in all our affairs.

Adapted and reprinted with permission of A.A. World Services, Inc.

The Twelve Traditions of Cocaine Anonymous

1. Our common welfare should come first; personal recovery depends upon C.A. unity.
2. For our group purpose there is but one ultimate authority—a loving God as He may express Himself in our group conscience. Our leaders are but trusted servants; they do not govern.
3. The only requirement for C.A. membership is a desire to stop using cocaine and all other mind-altering substances.
4. Each group should be autonomous except in matters affecting other groups or C.A. as a whole.
5. Each group has but one primary purpose—to carry its message to the addict who still suffers.
6. A C.A. group ought never endorse, finance or lend the C.A. name to any related facility or outside enterprise, lest problems of money, property, and prestige divert us from our primary purpose.
7. Every C.A. group ought to be fully self-supporting, declining outside contributions.
8. Cocaine Anonymous should remain forever nonprofessional, but our service centers may employ special workers.
9. C.A., as such, ought never be organized; but we may create service boards or committees directly responsible to those they serve.
10. Cocaine Anonymous has no opinion on outside issues; hence the C.A. name ought never be drawn into public controversy.
11. Our public relations policy is based on attraction rather than promotion; we need always maintain personal anonymity at the level of press, radio, and films.
12. Anonymity is the spiritual foundation of all our Traditions, ever reminding us to place principles before personalities.

Adapted and reprinted with permission of A.A. World Services, Inc.

The Twelve Steps Of Narcotics Anonymous

1. We admitted we were powerless over our addiction, that our lives had become unmanageable.
2. We came to believe that a Power greater than ourselves could restore us to sanity.
3. We made a decision to turn our will and our lives over to the care of God *as we understood Him*.
4. We made a searching and fearless moral inventory of ourselves.
5. We admitted to God, to ourselves, and to another human being the exact nature of our wrongs.
6. We were entirely ready to have God remove all these defects of character.
7. We humbly asked Him to remove our shortcomings.
8. We made a list of all persons we had harmed, and became willing to make amends to them all.
9. We made direct amends to such people wherever possible, except when to do so would injure them or others.
10. We continued to take personal inventory and when we were wrong promptly admitted it.
11. We sought through prayer and meditation to improve our conscious contact with God *as we understood Him*, praying only for knowledge of His will for us and the power to carry that out.
12. Having had a spiritual awakening as the result of these steps, we tried to carry this message to addicts, and to practice these principles in all our affairs.

Adapted and reprinted with permission of A.A. World Services, Inc.

THE TWELVE TRADITIONS OF NARCOTICS ANONYMOUS

1. Our common welfare should come first; personal recovery depends upon N.A. unity.
2. For our group purpose there is but one ultimate authority—a loving God as He may express Himself in our group conscience. Our leaders are but trusted servants; they do not govern.
3. The only requirement for N.A. membership is a desire to stop using.
4. Each group should be autonomous except in matters affecting other groups or N.A. as a whole.
5. Each group has but one primary purpose—to carry its message to the addict who still suffers.
6. An N.A. group ought never endorse, finance or lend the N.A. name to any related facility or outside enterprise, lest problems of money, property, and prestige divert us from our primary purpose.
7. Every N.A. group ought to be fully self-supporting, declining outside contributions.
8. Narcotics Anonymous should remain forever nonprofessional, but our service centers may employ special workers.
9. N.A., as such, ought never be organized; but we may create service boards or committees directly responsible to those they serve.
10. Narcotics Anonymous has no opinion on outside issues; hence the N.A. name ought never be drawn into public controversy.
11. Our public relations policy is based on attraction rather than promotion; we need always maintain personal anonymity at the level of press, radio, and films.
12. Anonymity is the spiritual foundation of all our Traditions, ever reminding us to place principles before personalities.

Adapted and reprinted with permission of A.A. World Services, Inc.

The Twelve Steps Of Alcoholics Anonymous

1. We admitted we were powerless over alcohol—that our lives had become unmanageable.
2. Came to believe that a Power greater than ourselves could restore us to sanity.
3. Made a decision to turn our will and our lives over to the care of God *as we understood Him.*
4. Made a searching and fearless moral inventory of ourselves.
5. Admitted to God, to ourselves, and to another human being the exact nature of our wrongs.
6. Were entirely ready to have God remove all these defects of character.
7. Humbly asked Him to remove our shortcomings.
8. Made a list of all persons we had harmed, and became willing to make amends to them all.
9. Made direct amends to such people wherever possible, except when to do so would injure them or others.
10. Continued to take personal inventory and when we were wrong promptly admitted it.
11. Sought through prayer and meditation to improve our conscious contact with God *as we understood Him*, praying only for knowledge of His will for us and the power to carry that out.
12. Having had a spiritual awakening as the result of these steps, we tried to carry this message to alcoholics, and to practice these principles in all our affairs.

Reprinted with permission of A.A. World Services, Inc.

The Twelve Traditions Of Alcoholics Anonymous

1. Our common welfare should come first; personal recovery depends upon A.A. unity.
2. For our group purpose there is but one ultimate authority—a loving God as He may express Himself in our group conscience. Our leaders are but trusted servants; they do not govern.
3. The only requirement for A.A. membership is a desire to stop drinking.
4. Each group should be autonomous except in matters affecting other groups or A.A. as a whole.
5. Each group has but one primary purpose—to carry its message to the alcoholic who still suffers.
6. An A.A. group ought never endorse, finance or lend the A.A. name to any related facility or outside enterprise, lest problems of money, property, and prestige divert us from our primary purpose.
7. Every A.A. group ought to be fully self-supporting, declining outside contributions.
8. Alcoholics Anonymous should remain forever nonprofessional, but our service centers may employ special workers.
9. A.A., as such, ought never be organized; but we may create service boards or committees directly responsible to those they serve.
10. Alcoholics Anonymous has no opinion on outside issues; hence the A.A. name ought never be drawn into public controversy.
11. Our public relations policy is based on attraction rather than promotion; we need always maintain personal anonymity at the level of press, radio, and films.
12. Anonymity is the spiritual foundation of all our Traditions, ever reminding us to place principles before personalities.

Reprinted with permission of A.A. World Services, Inc.

Cocaine Anonymous
P.O. Box 1367
Culver City, CA 90232
(213) 559-5833

Narcotics Anonymous
P.O. Box 9999
Van Nuys, CA 91409
(818) 780-3951

Alcoholics Anonymous
P.O. Box 459
Grand Central Station
New York, NY 10163
(212) 686-1100